The
Last
Hello

99 Odes
to the Body

D1293702

The
Last
Hello

99 Odes
to the Body

Joe Numbers

atmosphere press

Table of Contents

Oftentimes the things that

are closest to us

are the most difficult

to see.

Ode to the Feet

Our ancient
    fins have
evolved into our new
    five-toed
        wings:
you became the reason we can now travel
        beyond all known borders,
above and below our earthly plane,
        intricate
bundle of
    many bones,
odd bones, bones long and short.
Together you
push the
    moon-bound
        pedals.
Transient guest
of uncountable shoes,
some remembered,
some painfully not.

Our
        personal printmaker
you explain
        our mobile existence
        to the doubters:
quiet and methodical
        in your eternal pursuit
            of distance.
You become the cryptic witness
we leave behind
        in the sand
    to mark the
    insistence of
        our lives,
the necessity of our days:
that yes, indeed, we exist –
if only we return
    after the next

wave.
And occasionally
        we do.
We dance,
        you and I,
and we dance well.
And this is our agreement,
        our mutual
                celebration of this delicate
and occasionally clumsy life.

Platforms:
        personal,
                pliable,
                        improbable vehicles;
subject to occasional breakdowns
                and numerous detours
on our journey to somewhere
        once desired
                from our distant past.
Too many detours
                to count at this point.
                And the count continues.
You have this
        intimate knowledge
                of arches,
        fallen and otherwise.
And, yes,
        bunions,
                corns,
                        and the other pedestrian calamities
are the occasional normal.
        And I can live with that.

Your face is unique
        for each of us:
        all of your ridges and valleys
that add up to
        our personal blueprint;
        our unique upside-down signature.
I believe a fragile copy
        of mine resides in a dusty field

4

     somewhere north of here,
or perhaps it was many miles
     to the south.
But we can do so much more as you and I both know.
And we
   can do no
      better.

We dance!

Ode to the Toes

Thong-grippers
    and sand-
        sifters
for
half the world,
    for half the time.
Pink-eyed
    sardines
canned in leather
for most of
    the rest of us.

You curl,
you dig,
    you lift,
you wriggle.

Wriggle.
    Wriggling.
Something toes, apparently,
    do quite well.

You assist in our
    daily balancing act,
holding us steady
as we journey
to mostly familiar,
but occasionally strange places,
and then stranger memories.
You plot our
    nautical course;
        somewhere between
believable and, perhaps,
        something we've made up
and then shared –
    but only with
    our loved ones and other
        strangers.

Eager collector of
unmentionable
    jams
that we won't discuss
    in polite company or
    those other less casual settings.

Somewhere in time
someone started calling you
        little piggy's.
How did that happen?
Is this something you'd like
            to discuss?

You are the far
        southern fingers of our life;
a place we often need
        a passport to explore,
        and, more often,
                    to explain.
Did we ever decide on a name
            for your exotic realm?
    I think some day we definitely should.

Short, blunt and,
always
            to the point - at least when I'm paying
            attention.
    Maybe you're different
            in my dreams.
        Maybe not.
Maybe it depends on when I look at you
or the phase of the moon,
        or some other
                nocturnal event.

And yet you sift sand so well
        as I happily recall
from long-ago journeys -
some of them to paradise.
And some on the way back.

I trim your nails when I can;
when I have the stamina to reach
that far.
              And you appreciate it.
Shoes fit so much better when I do.

And did I mention that you curl?

Ode to the Left Little Toe

You represent the
    smallest extension
and the furthest
        conception
of who
I am.

Sometimes I forget you –
but occasionally
we do meet in person.
And when
    we do
I pretend
    not to notice you.
So you tease me – and rightfully so,
as if you were
    a ragged orphan,
abandoned by an
uncaring
        parent –
alone in your anatomic distance -
like an undiscovered
        planet circling an
unknown sun.

But you're not mean
about it.
And you know
    I really do care.
I think of you as my
    frontier outpost:
camping out so far away,
 keeping guard,
so close to the border,
so close to the edge of our
        corporeal boundaries.

You face the worst
of my fears on

a daily basis.
You touch the unknown -
and you do so
without flinching,
        without complaint.
You have been more brave
        than me so many times;
and my life is so much
        richer because of you.
Your desire to move forward
        is epic –
you are my brave Columbus
        in white socks
        and tennis shoes –
sailing the high seas –
        and occasionally
discovering
        foreign countries.

Closer to home,
and from where I stand,
you reside as far away
        as I can travel
and still be
        me.

Ode to the Soles of the Feet

You quietly became the
        prime witness
of our pedestrian lives,
and the silent outline
        of our passing
in these
    fragile times —
until the next wave
                washes in
        of course.

The
    thick and
        the thin,
the tough
and the ticklish,
the arbiter
of our working days
and the many small journeys
we string together
to tell the story
            of our life:
our quiet necklace
of purpose
        so to speak.

Your most recent life:
our personal interpreter
        of the earth's dirt
                and dust,
        and the ocean's infinite sand.
You have intimate
            knowledge of
and the various
natural and unnatural
            materials
that define our paths —
our daily journeys —
chosen or,

sometimes not.

Tactile
    navigator
from down south;
sailing entire continents
    by touch alone.
You know best
    of anyone
what our standing in
this world is.
You wear the shoes
    we choose
to name our lives with –
    if we're lucky –
because sometimes
    we don't have that choice.

You touch
    our daily truths
in simple or profound ways
    and yet you ask
      so little
        in return.
Many times
    we forget to thank you
      at the end of the day.
Intrepid and faithful
    companion,
you have been with us
    every step
      of the way.

Ode to the Ball of the Foot

Knuckle,
knob,
knot
tendon,
      bone, and
             flesh;
blunt edge
      of the articulated knife
that is
      our foot.

Drawbridge,
      springboard
and launching pad,
pivotal point
          of our departures,
keeper of our current momentum,
      the home of interesting and,
      as yet,
          un-named aches.
You intimately
live our daily travels.
You leave the deepest mark
on our longest journeys.

You
measure our shoes
      all by yourself,
at least that's what they tell me
at the shoe store.
      Maybe they know
          something I don't.
      And, of course,
          you're not talking.

You launch
      our today's
from the moment
      we arise,

and you launch our tomorrows,
        when we finally get to them,
when life permits,
        when you and our bones
and our muscles
all agree
that,
    yes,
        on this particular day,
           we have decided to
           go forward.

We have decided
      to begin
         again.

Ode to the Instep

Pale one,
>> our delicate stirrup,
the pink sail
of our nautical vessel,
>> you're at home on
>>> the high seas
>> and have intimate knowledge
>>>> of our most recent
>>>>> currents.
You begin and
>>> end
in the middle
>> of somewhere,
going someplace,
>>> somehow,
spanning small
>>> distances yourself,
and only a step
behind our dreams.
The ones that
take us home
occasionally,
>> but often,
>>> many miles beyond,
to those red, green, blue, and yellow
countries on the map,
>>> the big map,
the one too heavy to carry
>>> in our backpack.
The one we study
>> when we're
>>> back home
>> from our travels.
>>> Again.
>>>> And once more.

Suspended
between two piers
>>> of bone and muscle –

tender,
    ticklish,
        and sometimes –
when we dally too long in the tub –
 wrinkled belly
of our travels.
The travels we take,
sometimes in the light of day,
      sometimes not,
           no matter what
              time it is.

Inverted parachute
      of our best
          intentions,
and occasionally
the intentions we learned from
           our parents –
    whether we wanted to or not.

Tired bookkeeper
of our daily grind,
and the status quo of Mondays –
the ones that pay
the everyday bills,
and,
    occasionally,
           the ones that
           make a difference.

The ones we make
when we become intoxicated
    with the infinite possibilities
      this small blue planet presents,
you know,
    the ones that fit
      your soft and very particular
          curve.

Ode to the Heels

You became
    the first of me
to touch this earth,
and –
all things
    being equal –
the first to
    leave as well.

Calloused and rough,
and far too proud
for your own good,
you were born wrinkled
    and bald,
and you have made no effort to change –
    and so you remain.

Always taking it
    on the chin,
        so to speak,
and coming back
    for more
    you rarely complain.

    Prizefighter,
        our blue collar avatar:
you know
all of our pedestrian rules
    and can list them by name;
you have personally counted the mileage
    of our lives,
    some soft,
        and some hard,
some quick, slow, cautious or bold,
as if destiny,
    magic –
        and perhaps a little luck –
were the cosmic keys
    to where we will sleep anew tonight.

I think this has something
        to do with choices –
                but I could be wrong.

You continue to navigate
        our personal seas,
        always ready and
                always knowing -
because we
                passed this way before.

You,
having grown from innocent desire
                into bone and stubborn flesh,
will now
    lead us
                into our next tomorrow
once more,
        and once more,
                again.

Ode to the Ankles

Our primary pivot –
    you pivot –
        and then we walk.
Horizontal hinge,
I've heard a rumor that you are
the main reason
    that we walk
        upright:
you are at the heart
    of the matter
        so to speak.
You are the strategic command center
    of the foot:
        some kind
           of higher up
               down there.

Cotter pin,
    and toe tapper
        extraordinaire
content in your
    cocoon of skin and tendon,
there is, however, a certain
    rigidity in your
        interpretation
of what is,
and what is not, in those bounds –
and we have all
        paid
your particular
price
for crossing that line.

Yet you
    continue to walk these
    urban roads, these country roads,
these occasional beaches
and these many pilgrim trails with me,
    knowing full well that

so many
      have been wrong turns,
         blind alleys,
and yes,
      the occasional road to perdition
or something beyond.
And, yes, we often agree that –
      someone should have
          put a sign up
           a long time ago.

We continue,
and you allow,
we dream,
      and you permit,
we push the limits,
        and you provide the means.

We rest –
      on the left side of midnight –
      and that is when
         you prepare
for our departure
        at dawn.
That is when
      you read
        the map.

Ode to the Achilles Tendon

Tucked quietly
    into the back of our heels,
    and the back of our minds,
you have become the stern master
    of our daily movement,
the elastic lever
    of our primal fulcrum:
a glistening
    silver strand
        of pure fiber
        and living steel.

Broad and narrow
    by turns,
functional
    and yet fragile,
we shield you
from injury
    when we can.
But then,
    late at night,
when you are sleeping
and mostly unaware,
    we draw up our
newest adventures,
our latest reachings,
    and those distant flags
we have decided to explore –
usually without consulting you.

In fact we rarely think
    of you
and your fragile relation with
    such things as running,
        jumping, climbing, hiking
until it's too late –
and then we quickly review
    our recent actions
        and our

                    casual carelessness
toward you
        in minute and painful
                    detail.

Stretching and
        contracting,
more or less constantly,
you are the red-blooded laborer
            of our daily stride.
You were born
        in practicality,
dedicated to
        achieving sometimes small
and sometimes worldly
            distances,
often in small steps
        and occasionally in
                great leaps.
It helps
        that you are so
                patient.

Married to our southern bones
        in mysterious ways,
you direct our daily world
            of motion and distance
in obvious ways,
and, when you can -
        you help us set things right.

When morning arrives,
we arise and
        we task you again
                with our velocity,
direction, purpose
and those distant flags.

And we drink
        from the silver chalice
        of your singular purpose.
The purpose you spoke of –

late last night.
And then you remind us
that we spoke once again
             of movement
        when dawn finally arrives.

        And so we did.
                And so we begin anew.

Ode to the Calves

Stride makers,
rising from
      behind
yet pushing us
          forward;
from times faintly
          remembered,
to places often
          unknown
and finally
          back home.
You are the reason
      we can move
      from room to room,
      from city to city,
from green familiar countryside to
          dry foreign deserts:
      the Atacama
          comes to mind.

Twin-headed cobra,
      bundle of eager muscles
          and directional magic,
sleek and supple,
      taut and rigid,
slender and stout
      by turns,
you guide us
      into the day,
and then,
      on to the night.
And we trust you:
      you are the conductor
          of our erotic desires:
you get us there,
you take us to our
      midnight destinations
      and the many way-stations
          in-between.

Jump masters,
       toe dancers,
basketball and
          ballet
are two of your biggest challenges;
       your shining moments
             of fame and stardom,
these are the contests
         you adore
            the most.
And for the rest of us –
       we can always dream.

Through you
       we can even fly,
un-bound,
       immortal,
          briefly,
              briefly,
and back to earth.
       And then we continue
       our daily encounter with gravity.

And tomorrow,
       as always,
we await the new day's journey,
and you,
       as always,
eager
to devour the miles,
like the hungry cheetah
       that you are,
chasing, pouncing and then catching
our usual prey:
       distance –
         as always,
           by the end
              of the day.

Ode to the Shinbone

Here is
        the leading edge
of our lower
                aeronautical lives,
our solid strut and
        landing gear,
leaving the
        runway
in small
        increments,
rise, flight, glide and return,
you are the seasoned pilot
of our daily commute -
ready to take off
        on our slightest command –
our pilot of sorts
        you lead the daily charge
Here is the
        tibial scythe
of our agricultural lives
cutting a
        silver path
                ever wider,
                        ever longer,
        through the ripe and golden fields of
our expectant lives;
you help us reap the many rewards
        of our daily dreams.

Shiny prow
        of our nautical lives,
cutting through our everyday oceans,
our sometimes calm
        and
        our sometimes stormy seas.
You are keenly aware of the lighthouses
        on those distant rocky shores,
        guiding us safely
to our destinies -

and then home again.
And, hopefully,
                again,

Our knobbed and sturdy walking stick,
                burled bone,
fearless pathfinder,
you lead the way -
                whether you like it or not.
I can't even count
how many times you have
found silent bedposts,
misplaced treasures -
                and other immovable objects -
                                in the dark;
some vertical,
                some horizontal -
                                and always sudden.

I patch you up
                often,
and then you go and volunteer again -
                and I'll never understand why.
We should have
                a discussion sometime —
                at your convenience,
                                of course.

But this is what I do understand
with the clear voice that
                you declared long ago:
We shall walk!
                And yes,
                                thanks to you,
                                                we do.

Ode to the Kneecaps

Looking like
        a cross
between the full moon
and a
        buffalo skull,
mounted on the
        leading edge
of our knee like a
        blind navigator,
like a figurehead
        of sorts,
        and mostly of the
                nautical kind.
You are the brave
        forerunner,
our shield of solid bone,
our collector
        of a thousand
childhood
        mishaps.
Sidewalks and
        second bases,
backyards and playing fields
all have
        intimate knowledge
of the kneecap,
where earth, sky, and tendons
come together
        and call themselves
                horizon.

You are the front line of our mobile defenses,
        our warrior of the midnight unknown.
Many times
you are the first to land in
        our forward assault
                on the sandy beaches
                        of gravity.
And other less friendly

                    places.
And we are
        grateful for
                your bravery,
both voluntary and
                accidental.
We've been meaning
        to send you
                a thank you note.

Small distant butte
        of white stone,
often a perfect stranger,
always quiet and unassuming,
        until we meet again,
and usually
        when we
                least expect it.
You make your presence known,
        and when you insist –
                        we listen.

Pale outcropping
        of bone
shimmering quietly
                in the moonlight,
somewhere between pleasure
                and pain;
the quick
        and the dead;
and always
                about
                        halfway
                        to the ground.

Sitting or standing
        your status is
                never in doubt –
and we always know
                when you have
                something more to say.

Ode to the Knees

Not really
    a clean break,
but you are still anatomically
                correct,
and obviously in the right location.
Our complicated
and sometimes fragile
                        gift,
you give us
such everyday miracles as:
forward
        and backward,
sitting and
        kneeling,
running and
        jumping,
                among many others,
    usually more than I
                    can count.
After all is said and done –
        you are the reason
            we keep diaries.

Bony outpost of
        pure movement,
your purpose
        always lies
just around
                the next corner
        and the latest explanation.
You have so many surfaces
        that I have lost count –
but occasionally I feel
                every single one.

Always the friend
  of our
        curious souls,
you propel us to
our next destination,

occasionally without
our permission
or forethought –
but always wanting
            to please.

Fortress of bone
        and tendon,
        ligament and muscle
you express endless
                movement –
until suddenly,
            you don't.

At times we
        stand directly on top of you.
For example:
when we tend to
            our green gardens,
when we have
        face-to-face conversations
                with sad four-year old's,
and when we
        need to make peace
            with our many gods.

Occasional stick breaker,
        we use you
as a living fulcrum
when our fragile hands alone
        cannot accomplish
            the job.
You often complain,
        but always comply
with our occasional
                whims.

You have become one of the many
wonders
        of the human form:
just ask any
        penguin.

Ode to the Thighs

Sturdy pillars,
by turns
soft and
       translucent,
       hard and muscular,
       athletic – or not,
and always vulnerable to the vagaries
             of our next destination.

You are often lit from
           within,
by some inner flame,
       from some mysterious origin -
           with an unpronounceable name.
Twin roots of our
       singular bodies –
extending from somewhere
       below the waist to
       somewhere above the knee –
as if you alone
       own that entire region.
               And so you do.

You are the foundation
       of our southern strength;
our ally in the many trenches of our
           everyday lives.
You are the spawning bed
       of our earthly desires,
the supple storehouse
       of our
           sexual dreams.

You can be the color of
       honey
           or cream or onyx.
You begin, live
       and end where pure
           motion resides,
where pure passion rules,

where reason has little meaning.
You claim this as
        your rightful home,
                your femoral kingdom
and we can only agree
                to this earthly arrangement.

All muscle, direction
        and purpose,
you push
        and pull
our daily burdens:
some light,
        some heavy
        and some our fleeting pleasures.
You treat them all
        equally.
You withhold judgement,
        and
        your intentions are
                always innocent.

Rippling, incandescent
                thighs.
You often announce your
        innocence
of these worldly matters,
but we know better.
You have been there
        our entire lives.
        You have seen
                everything.

Ode to the Testicles

Occasionally you act as
    the center of the
        universe —
the star of the show -
        however briefly you shine.
Mostly though,
you are the pale outliers
of our human evolution,
partially hidden
    among the pubic reeds
somewhere along the
        southern border.

You react to our
        erotic desires
in predictable ways
when they occur,
and then you scheme constantly
    to make sure they come true.
And you are keenly aware
        of your importance:
You supply the purpose,
    the meaning and
        the end result
of our primal will to survive.
We rarely comment
    on your relentless drive -
but you persist
in your own way.
    Like a living phoenix
        you return to the ultimate
          scene:
the warm and humid reproductive spring
that calls to us
after a long winter
        without solace.

Birthplace of dreams,
and frequent calls to glory,
you are the

living storehouse of our family's history
nestled in your
        leathery, wrinkled, and air-conditioned pouch –
your thick and thin pouch –
depending on circumstances -
        which are
                rarely within your control.

Miniature miracle factories
and birthplace
of a billion spontaneous sperm,
you still see the world
        in simple terms:
create life,
        always more life,
and always in your mirror image –
like the jealous little demi-gods
                that you are.

Are you the determined pilots
        of our impetuous and often short
                                lives?
Or are you
        merely the hijacked passengers
        on our occasionally
                dangerous flights of desire?
We know for certain that
        the concept of consequences
        rarely, if ever, enters into
                your midnight equations.
When passion calls
        you are always
                eager to answer
        in you singular way –
                tomorrow be damned.

In the end,
        we know that your sole purpose
in life is
simply to correspond
                with distant ovaries -
your identical twins

from an earlier life.
And you exchange postcards
              at every opportunity.

Ode to the Penis

Blunt instrument of desire,
one-eyed delivery man
                    of sorts,
            you are like a
            heat-seeking missile
searching for your
                    clitoral twin
            from a previous life
and the primal warmth
you remember
            within an otherwise
                    cold and
                            uncaring world.

You seem to live a
                    dual life
            with a dual purpose:
constantly changing your silhouette
to accommodate
            the most pressing of our needs –
whether they are necessary or not -
and occasionally without our permission.
            You come and go
                    as they say.

You consist of
            many parts:
a singular anchor,
            multiple anatomical columns,
and finally the stoic face
            you present
                    to the world.
Evacuation and ejaculation
            are the essential verbs
            that define your
                    earthly existence.
This is your high-wire
                    trapeze act,
perfected over the millennia:
you tend to seek balance -

and occasionally
you find it.
Photos never do
you justice,
since you are rarely
in focus –
although you often leave
tracks –
some subtle,
some enigmatic –
and others hidden
in plain sight.
Some of your tracks
are temporary and
pass quickly
with the melting snow;
others are more permanent,
easily outlasting our singular lives -
and for many
generations beyond.

I'd like to think
you take full
ownership
of everything you do –
but we know that
is rarely true.
Just another myth
on top of your
mountain of myths –
dating back to ancient times,
or perhaps not:
for starters it turns out that your
size and circumference
are based mostly on
who's telling
the story.

You appear to live in
a parallel universe
with your female counterparts:
you share so much history

neatly folded into
        your many components –
your primordial beginnings.
You also occasionally share
        volcanic eruptions
in your mutual attempts
        to create new islands
in the sea of human life.

Apparently, you are
        never satisfied with
                the status quo.

Ode to the Vagina

Beneath the
delicate vulvar crown,
        a pale rose emerges from
        those soft pillows,
moist and sweet,
always with your singular
                promise of heaven
                        on earth –
and you lead us on -
                and then you lead us onward.

Protected by
        the labial shield,
soft bay of personal
                solitude,
moody like the sea -
        you ebb and
                flow,
gently –
        or not.

        Harbor,
                harbor,
                        harbor.

Delicate portal,
        muscular portal,
genital doorway to our
        past, present and future.
        Mysterious keyhole,
you keep
        life's secrets
                locked safely within your
                mysterious depths,
and, in due time,
        your secrets emerge.
Some of them are perfect –
                and others come with
                        a more complex
                                story to tell.

You are a sometimes reluctant host,
        a hungry connoisseur of
                both pleasure and intrigue -
        with only a passing interest
                in today's news -
but we know you are
                always keeping score.
Because of you
        we are also always counting.
And when we reach
        the lunar boundary of
                your existence —
we start counting -
                again and then again.

Sometimes you listen to
        our shared emotions —
even though
it is hard for you to admit —
as all the centuries
        behind us will confirm.
You have been
the origin of many wars -
        most of them small,
                        short,
                        and very local.
Others have involved
        jealous nations and
        untold myths and odysseys -
                according to the history books.
Would you agree?

Your physical costumes
        appear to be endless.
You set the stage
in your singular
        and intimate way.
And the actors
        appear as if
                by magic —
and strut

                   their sometimes brief,
and tragic
         hour upon your
                   fertile stage.

You lead somewhere,
and you know the
                   way,
you are the guide
that points us
         to eternity —
or the redemption
                   of hope —
         whichever comes sooner.

You are the
         hidden beauty
of human life.
         We exist because
                   you exist.
But this has
         never been a simple
                   transaction.

Ode to the Ovaries

Aviaries.
        miniature
                bird cage
                of our human life.
The cage where
        our dreams begin.

One at a time,
        small delicate creatures
                take flight
        from within your exotic confines —
and then migrate -
        when they can -
                along your southern
                                coast
to a rendezvous
        with their
                eager counterparts,
the lucky ones,
        the persistent ones,
the ones with
        nothing to lose -
        at least not for tonight.

If only it were
        that simple.

Eggs are born within you —
        and how is that even possible?
Eggs getting born?
        Is this the storied tent
        in the desert
where miracles
        suddenly occur?

Flanking the northern
        reaches of the uterus —
you are on intimate terms with
        the fallopian tubes —
our earth-bound passage ways

to glory
          or despair,
or,
more often,
          somewhere in between.

You are the
          deep well of our sexual essence:
you control the
          cycles of desire,
the urgency,
and the sudden future
          of so many soon-to-be lives.

Symmetrical spheres
          of fertility –
each of you apparently
has an equal say
          in the ultimate equation:
You watch the calendar,
          you watch the days -
                    and you never lose
                              track of your primitive count.

You maintain your
          spherical perfection
in spite of the
          multiple assaults
                    on your intimate castle:
Your moat is
          just deep enough.

And finally,
          you always
                    have the last word.

Ode to the Womb

There is
  within each of us
the struggle
  to reach for
      light,
  to reach for life
and you are the place
    and the home
    where it all begins.
And yes, we
do look back
    from the moment
      we leave,
at the infinite
    paradise
    that you are,
the personal
    green house,
the storied garden
    of our immediate past.

The most mysterious
    and the most precious
of the organs,
riding there unseen
    between the hips
giving hope to
our choices,
and the life we have
        chosen.

Temporary waiting room,
    and terrestrial rehearsal space
    before we make
our once-in-a-lifetime
            appearance.

Finicky organ,
    filling with
    blood once

45

a month
    in anticipation,
rising with
    the tide,
    and your lunar schedule.
The promise of
a future birth —
    always within reach.

The mad scientist
of our personal lives.
You combine our
    genetic chemicals
with such
    precision
that we hesitate
    to call it
        a science;
it is that far
    beyond our mortal grasp.

While your
    belly swells
    with life,
my love,
mine swells
    with pride,
and you,
    swollen miracle,
I can touch you,
    I can see you,
        I can feel you.
and I can believe in you:
the circle
    that completes
        the circle of life.

You conjure the origin,
    the alpha and the omega.
Without you,
    there is no beginning
        and no end.

Ode to the Pubic Hair

Gathered together into a
bed of
soft reeds,
like a song
      of intent,
a flourish,
an unrehearsed symphony
      of many individual notes
brought to life,
and then you begin;
        a chorus
that we have all heard
        from the beginning.

A field lying naked
      in the spring
is still a future
        promise,
an unexplained
      desire
to know more;
and then,
      the sorcery begins:
innocence trades
      places with fertility,
      fantasy with virility,
the lioness makes
      her home,
the lion launches
      his legacy.

An outward chronicle of our years,
our individual story
      of roots, textures
        and proportions.
Nest of small, damp
        lightening
you lie at the confluence
      of desire and destiny,
an amorous river

of eddies and currents,
a mysterious map
to be explored,
perhaps with compass in hand.

Triangular shield of transparent modesty,
the
            beginning of
our intimate fantasies,
the tangled treasure
              we seek
                      in our nightly dreams.

Ode to the Buttocks

Cloud burst of
      muscle and flesh,
paired whales
beneath the
      waves of our
      restless belts;
a multiple of geography
      in motion,
the public showcase
      of our various ways
      and various means:
our intimate history –
      and how we got here.

Seashells
      of erotic softness,
plunging and rising
with your unique brand
        of symmetry
like epic waves
      breaking somewhere west
of the pubic
      archipelago.

Hidden yet
      continuous beauty,
you lie in
      waiting.
You steal the
      show
whenever you can –
      and that's quite often
      by my count at least.

You propel us forward
      with every breath.
Every step is made
      in your name.

Primal cleavage,

your silence is legendary,
yet for something
so quiet,
you speak multiple volumes.

Your moves
write sensual novels
in my mind.

Ode to the Anus

You lie staunchly at anchor below
                    like some muscular
                                    ring of elimination,
the gateway of
our never-ending
                    stream of refuse
and the site of our
            often scented attempts
at cleanliness
when we are done.

You live quietly
            and with singular purpose —
while your erogenous
            qualities lie
            veiled and
                        unknown
in most conversations.
And you can easily judge
            our lives based
on what does - or doesn't -
                        pass your way.

Circle of infamy,
            and subject of countless jokes
serving us efficiently
in your simplicity,
like a naked moth
nearing the
            candle,
the sudden fluttering
of your pale
                        wings,
the blinking of an unseeing eye,
the hasty signing
            of final papers,
and then you return again
            to the darkness;
the rising eclipse

of another day
to mark your daily existence.

Ode to the Pelvic Bone

Windswept and slender
      iceberg of bone,
      floating amid
           the equatorial
                regions,
the abdominal depths;
our
    bridge of life,
      the natal shield,
delineator of the
      meridional dimensions.

Conform to the
rigid geometry
from which we suspend our
latest fashions,
our rainbows,
      our supply of many belts,
      like birds of prey landing
      on our anatomical shore,
like eagles frozen in
          mid-stroke.
Winged deposit of calcium
      and movement –
with your pierced ears
and determined attitude:
you look like an
    angel
      about
         to land.

You know intimately the place
where the muscles
      of our intentional motion
gather and finally
    come home to roost,
    the landing place
      of our femurs
      and the foreign destinations
that we dream about

on a daily basis —
the ones you help us reach
                         when you can.
You give anatomical structure
            to the idea of motion —
definitely
            not an easy task — but one
you supply with
            an abundance of grace
            and occasional caution.

Bony butterfly,
            you come in many parts —
                        a trilogy of sorts.
The ossified shovel
of our lust and fertility,
            our pubic guardian,
and the unheralded champion of athletes:
and the reason
            human speed records exist -
            and that we can never get enough.

You have intimate relations
            with the sacrum
                        on a daily basis —
something no one thought possible.
You appear to be
                        always listening —
hearing our pleas
                        and complaints,
supporting our joys
                        and pleasures,
            our travels and temptations.

Whenever you can,
and whenever we let you,
you deliver our
                        destinations.

Ode to the Tailbone

The fossilized homage
        of our
        ancestral image,
the mirror we look
                back on our beginnings with,
our hidden lineage,
tucked neatly between
        the buttocks.
You quietly announce the last
                segment
of the vestigial tail,
the last chapter
        of our family history –
                so to speak.
Short as a thumb
and older than
        memory itself;
there was a time,
so many eons ago,
        that you were
our whole substance:
a tail
        and two eyes
emerging from
        the primordial
                lagoon.

And now
        a small reminder,
a flickering candle
        of bone,
a common
        coat-of-arms,
our fifth limb now lost
        to the whims
                of evolution.
Something we had
        little say in –
but that's probably
        for the best.

in this particular scheme
                              of things.

You write the latest edition
            of an ancient script –
a record written in
            common minerals
            with an uncommon ending.

Opaque finger
            of the ancient past,
you point downward
when we are upright,
the missing link,
the alpha
            and omega
                        of a million years
of living history.
Invisible and
all but forgotten –
sleeping contentedly
            in your Jurassic world.
A celebrity with
            a fading star,
you only come forward
            when we land
            upside down.
And that reminds us,
                        once again,
                                    not to forget you.

Ode to the Abdomen

Rising like a
vagabond moon,
above the
       pubic reeds,
now unfolding with
       our desires,
the
       anatomical balance
between intimate dimensions
and regional territories.
You reside in the
       in-between-land,
the land
       of crucial connections,
a most familiar land,
a land we can never abandon.

Wave maker,
       birthplace
              of our southern waves
       and sudden storms,
you are the quiet gatekeeper:
tightening
with our intentions and fears
or expanding
with our happy sighs
       and gastronomical successes.
Shielded by muscles
       you march continually
                  forward
in some quest for contentment –
no matter how humble
       or hopeful that might be.

You represent the
       home of
the miracle of digestion:
a living container
       holding our
       various and sundry organs in

some kind of
            purposeful arrangement.
Always pushing
        against gravity
            and our own vanity –
sometimes we win,
            and too often, we don't.
Apparently you reside at
        the home of mysterious buttons:
usually linked to
        past lives and long-forgotten lovers.

You constantly listen
        to our hunger
            or contentment –
with the ears
of a blind poet –
you talk often
and you amplify
        our abundance
        or the pain
            of its absence.

Ode to the Navel

Scar of the
       infinite past,
center of our
       living flesh,
moving with
       equatorial
              exactitude
in triumph
toward the
       final latitude;
       the latest haven.
   collector of
wind and tears,
intimate songs,
and the wine
       of love unleashed
            and prone.

Sleepless eye,
while you watch,
silent, prescient one,
we carry on
with our lives;
we the hopeful
and we who
are never
          satisfied.

Fountainhead,
mute rose of our
          personal beginnings,
mysterious footprint
       in the constantly changing sand,
like the faint echo
       of some
          past life.

Keeper of our
       deepest secrets,
and from you,
       we keep none.

Ode to the Small of the Back

I can only
know you directly
through mirrors,
               pain
                    and fatigue.
          Well-spring of
               flat steel
and tendon
          and most delicate
               of our curves,
and yet your name
          is written
on every monument,
          every statue
and every stone ever
          lifted to build
               an emerging world.

Spinal leaf,
          supple leaf,
in your hands
you carry the
          history of humans,
written in sharp
          darting pains
or the dull
          calligraphy
of sweat
          and grimace.

Small horizon,
and wanting the best
          of everything,
you bend
          and pull,
you rotate
and you span
          the gap.

Your essence
will always be unresolved,
         and always,
seeking the place
         you'd rather be.

Ode to the Spine

Cleaving the body
    like a petrified sword,
you measure the
    ultimate heights of our
        earthly growth.
As much as we'd like to,
    we cannot lie to you.

And we need you
    just to see that,
    bony sheath of
our biological lightening,
the ossified pathway of our
    sinuous
    and often savage
        voltage.

You also lead us to
the windows
    and gardens
of our eccentric
    planet.
And we indulge
    your offer
    when we can.

Staircase of
    our anatomical heritage,
you will continue to span
    the millenniums
as if you were
the bridge
    of human knowledge,
as if you were a
    midwife
to the dinosaurs
and then
    a short warning call
to the
    distant future.

Ode to the Nerves

Web of submerged
            lightening,
touching every
            nook and cranny
of our being
with fingers
            the size of
                        slender metal,
salt of our
            immediate response,
you both answer and
            call,
conjuring tears
            or laughter,
or barking
            like a black dog
at every intruder.

Blind map
            of our
            internal terrain,
translator,
            interpreter,
system of our systems;
when I speak
it is your
            bright rain
that answers,
and when I touch
            the doors
                        to paradise,
it is with
            your net
            flung madly into the
                        wind.

Ode to the Rib Cage

Sinking and
      rising
like a
mid-summer moon,
supple volume of
steadfast movement
      and human metronome,
you count our lives
with the
precision
      of a bony staircase.

You demonstrate both
the sequence
and the timeline
      of how we
      learned to
            capture the wind,
      of our breathless adoration
of time,
like the faraway awakening,
the turn
      and then the approach
of a sensual earthquake.

Anatomical chamber,
keeper of our
      many secrets,
home of the sternum
and living container
      of our vital organs —
the ones we can't
      live without.

Lattice of bone
      and breath,
cage of cartilage,
you with the infinite knowledge
      of our spine
            and our lengthy past

having to deal with gravity.

And,
              as you well know,
we share our long history
                      with the dinosaurs:
it was the same
              arrangement.

Ode to the Shoulders

Granite and
leaves
are your companions
as you travel
the structural regions
   and then the sensual regions
                  of our lives.
Pride
of structural engineers,
both ox,
         the mule,
and camel of
         our most recent
                  upright centuries,
you carry the
                  burden.
And promise to keep
                  your promise.

House of
familiar ways
and way-station
of the well-defined
         purpose.
And, yes, mostly
         you understand
                  my fleeting goals.

As of today
every sorrow
         ever recorded
                  has passed
over your subtle curves,
and you remember
         each of their faces,
and each of their names.

Gathering the fabric
of our lives
         into an

earthly symphony
of both tenderness
        and strength,
you deliver
the merchandise,
you deliver
what the
dream merchant sells,
and then you lift the
        world into view –
for the rest of us
                to see.

World of ligaments and
        muscles and tendons –
a marvel of pure art
                and architecture.
It is often said that
you carry the weight of
                the world –
which you occasionally embrace
                or deny -
depending on your mood
                and the time of day.
Your incredible range
                of movement
belies a delicacy
        you are reluctant
                to discuss.
But you always answer
        when I ask for your help.

Ode to the Shoulder Blades

Gilded wings,
        vestigial wings,
osseous plate
of pure
        geometry,
and base of our
        earthly reach:
What ancient paths
        did you take?
How many treasures
and easy answers
        did you leave
            behind
in order to
to build your
        aerie
on the back
        of humans?

You have become
        the hard
            landing
of so many muscles –
gathered to the
        idea of future
        and someday flight.
Arrowhead of bone,
        angel of movement,
            wings of our human
instincts and
        passing impulses,
you make both fantasy
        and reality come true.

Folded and flared
        like a rose petal
        lost in the garden
            of our bones,
you make the connection,
        you are the socket,

you make sense.

And when the nights
        touch the
                horizon ever so lightly:

Do you remember
        the names
of her hands?

Ode to the Chest

Lengthwise,
        a state of mind,
in width,
        an end in itself,
                masculine or
                feminine,
it doesn't really
        matter:
a breathing rock of ages,
        an earthbound balloon of sorts.

This is where
our central
muscles meet,
        face to face
in a mutual
        arrangement;
in constant motion,
in a perfect
        reflection of our
        current predicament.

Apparently you appear
        barrel-shaped on some,
        and sunken on others,
our mythical
        treasure chest:
the protector of our
        precious jewels —
        the ones we can't live
                        without.

In the beginning
        you spent all
        of your resources
becoming
a rhythmic,
interstellar cage,
        and in the end,
        you became

                    the hero
                            of heroes.

Breastplate
  of blood, ligament
                    and bone,
you protect the
            arterial labyrinth,
you provide the
            safe haven
            for our unknowable organs,
                        and their many secrets.

And, yes, you've seen it all.

Ode to the Breasts

Gentle ones,
you flood
    the night
with your
    volcanic curves,
with your call
    as soft as
the distant
    train whistle,
you bring the
    milk of swans
and other mythical creatures
    to our lives.
What happens next
    is mostly unique.

Motherhood re-incarnate and
    mysterious link
to so many
    other species;
we gladly share
    your name and purpose
    with so many
        unlike us.
There is a
    clandestine
        ripeness
within you,
ever green
ever the feeling
    of maternal
        spring.

Delicate crescent,
pale cup and
    the comfort
of humankind,
    - we are all born
        beneath your
            graceful shadow.

Unfolding rose,
both essence and
       fragrance,
we are your
       eager and hungry children.

Nautical arc,
       both wave and sea,
       ever welcome,
       always,
       and ever
               our most recent
                     history
                now explained.

Ode to the Nipples

The completed
       movement,
the symphony now
          at rest,
the mammary climax
and brief mooring
       of entire races and nations;
when I look at you
       I see both the
       ancient silhouette
and our future in waiting:
I believe that you are the one thing
       that we have all touched
          from the beginning..

Through your
       gentle eyes
flow the tears
       of humanity,
the pale honey
       of motherhood,
and all the bones
of those recently born.

In your touch:
       the first lessons of life,
the beginning
       of light,
the sweet halo
       of love gained
          and love given.

You pack an entire
          universe
       into a rose bud
       just waiting to bloom.
The point of beginning
       and the point of
          our departure;
       the last image

of our fleeting
        infancy.

You are
        the answer,
to our many questions,
and yet always:
        you are also
                the mirror.

Ode to the Arms

I have watched
you grow in
different lights,
and from many different sides.
Whenever I
        change shoes and hats
        you are waiting there:
        growing, veined,
        occasionally wounded,
        and always reaching.

I watch
from a short distance,
your treaties,
        your promises
of bright tomorrows,
the liquid facts,
        the meager rations
you assemble
        for my choices
during the day,
and the exotic dreams
you bring home at night.

And yet there
        is something
that eludes your grasp;
a note,
        a glance,
           an odor,
the return of a holy prophet
or the ancient proposition
        of human survival.

There is something
about you that is
        larger than life,
even larger than the body
        you sprang from –
        revered in ancient times

as one of the gods of our
          own body.

And you have
never failed me
whenever I have renewed
          that struggle;
with
          the unmistakable verbs
                    of touch,
the incredible communion
          of fingers
as they play my
          simple symphonies,
the theory of three
          that you still believe in,
the opaque moments you still proudly wear,
and the many scars of
          embracing
                    a world
made of
          narrow paths.

Ode to the Forearm

Being the lead note
        of a rainbow,
perhaps you've never
thought of honesty
as anything
        but a virtue –
and it shows.
Wearing a coat
        of round blue rivers,
tributaries and trinkets,
a few forgotten scars
                from childhood,
and the many ribbons and bands
                strapping time
tightly to your neck –
        as if you cared,
                as if you could care.

And you have endured.
You have always understood
        what was ahead,
no matter which
direction I chose;
and if I wrote a poem
        about someone
I have loved –
in between the hazy
grips of time
        and distance –
you would also understand.

Even if I told you
that she could heal
the bloodless wounds
                of love,
it would not
        surprise you.
That too,
is something you
        have always known.

Cylindrical,
          sculptural,
living between two extremes,
          aerodynamic in your
                    own strange way,
house of numerous muscles,
both large and small,
my strength is your kingdom,
          and the extension
                    I have always needed.

You allow me to reach
          for the nearest star —
for the love I
          have always sought,
and to reach back
for all the loves I have
          left along the wayside.
Are these quests the true purpose of my
          many wanderings?
Did you ever
          consider that?

Your honesty
                    has always been
                              beyond virtue.
And I, personally,
          have never questioned
                    your intentions.

That goes
          without saying.

Ode to the Armpits

Damp cave
        of muscle and skin
with your silken moss,
moist from our labors,
or shorn smooth
to please
the goddess
        of Vanity.

Local bridge of
        veins and arteries,
endless well
        of our personal
                essence,
tender amusement
                center,
and eternal butt of our cruelest
        jokes:
the one part
        of our bodies
        we try to
                forget –
        but then we are
                called back
        on a daily basis.

Fragrant nest of our
                personal pheromones –
and several other
                mysteries
we have yet
        to solve.

So here is your tribute:
you
    who deserves more,
you,
    who always
        knows our score,
this is it,

          armpit:
one bouquet of odors
and other intimate reminders
          to another –
and we always know
          when you are
                    winning.

Ode to the Muscles

Gathered sails
      leaning into
          the years,
lifter of eyelids
and the fibrous core
      of our every motion.

You drift unneeded
      for days –
and we risk
losing you;
this marriage, apparently, of
      alchemy and tendons
and the lessons of the road –
because nothing else can explain
      how you came
          to be.

You record the genius
of humankind without question,
and our passions
      without answer.
We are remembered because you
      continue to set records.

Written on the
thin paper of sudden reflexes,
you know the difference
      between life
      and the dark grey unknown.

From ditches to temples
nothing has been
      accomplished without
your mute consultation
and the unison of
      your glistening purpose;
the merging of your
slender red waves
with the ropes

and tools
of an
            unfinished world.
To the desert
            tortoise
you represent a precious
            patch of shade,
to the albatross –
            another hemisphere.

And we,
            the dreamers,
            the thieves
and the lovers,
we are
            no different
            in our desires.

Gambler,
you spin the
            very wheels
                        of our lives,
as if our fortunes
            depended on it.
You know the
            exact longitude
            and the fleeting odds
of our every movement.

Stairway of
            contractual stone,
breather of our breath,
you take the
            first step,
you understand the predominant
                                    chord
            of our singular symphony,
our kinetic theory,
the initial harvest
and finally,
            the end result.

Ode to the Elbows

Flash pan
of the un-named
        sensation,
table-top tripod
of un-followed
        dinner manners,
one-way crotch
of the upper
        landing gear
and a
        song flung
onto the beach
of our personal
                sea.

Yardstick —
we have used you
        to measure our world
        since the beginning of time.
Supple prop
        we use you
        to hold our weary
                heads up.
Backward facing —
        forward reaching hinge,
knob of wrinkled skin —
with few exceptions
        you have left
        your unique fingerprint
everywhere we have
                been.
And you have
        written it all down
in your rough language —
        the one we all
                learned long ago..

The applications
of your special arc
        are without limit,

your humor is
        flawless,
        unexpected
        and brilliant —
much like
        a flash of lightening.

Your hinge-like
qualities are,
        without doubt,
the final assurance
of your continuing
                existence,
a cause for
        celebration,
an occasion
without beginning
        or end.

Neural bend and
seismic sword
in crowded
        spaces,
you clear the way
you live at
        right angles
to the rest
of the
        anatomical world,
you attend concerts
on the edge
of perpetual
        motion —
and you understand
                every note.

Ode to the Wrists

Starting from
        an impulse,
and the desire to
        be complete,
the desire to extend beyond
our ancestral fins;
you were born
        to live in the future,
born to know
the day when
        thumbs, knuckles
                and fingers –
with your help of course –
would guide us
to the lunar mountains,
rolling back the
        very edges
of our heavens,
        and our hells –
and you were the
        connection –
you were
always the human connection.

And in softer times
you allow the
softness
        to become a caress.

There is a calmness
        to your many actions
and a confidence amid
the uncertainty
of fast approaching
        careers
        and then – suddenly –
                upcoming retirements.
Apparently,
        you take all this
                in stride.

You exceed
the limits of grace
        on a daily basis
without looking back.
And no one thought
that was even possible.

When I stand
in the middle
        of a crossroads,
I can hear your
        heartbeat from
                every direction –
        a triumph of
                spatial design.

You can be either the
        broad avenue
or the dusty
country road -
depending on who you
        tend to believe;
you weigh their
        gold or wheat
                with equal ease.

You bridge the
days of our lives
        like a hidden secret,
like a machine
arranging the sunsets,
        and, as always,
                dressed
                in many colors.

Ode to the Hands

We come to know you,
          one by one
carrying the
          fragile blueprints
of our lives
and we ask for
          your approval,
knowing that you
          will grant it
with a sly smile
          and then,
                    with many warnings.

A pure concept,
          on par
                    with the arms
and, much like the arms,
          a complete package.
A package
that we never saw
                    coming.
but we are grateful you did

And so we begin the lessons,
          you the teacher,
the owner of touch,
the mute carpenter
          of our visions,
the tool with which
          we pry open the locks.
You are both
the cup
                    and the sword –
and equally good
                    at both.

The piano exists
          because you exist.
Symphonies exist
          because you

also believe in harmony.

A description of
        your ridges,
valleys and peninsulas
is a major treatise:
        wars have been fought
                for less,
and then a gentle exchange
        of reluctant prisoners,
various rounded shapes
and something
        called purpose.

You are a theory
which can never
        be proven,
a brave
        answer
to the many claims of
                knowledge
        of this world,
and to those who
would deny the
existence of
architects,
        masons,
        musicians
                and the other magicians
                of the world.

I have never
        asked more
                from you
                than this.
And
you have always
        been enough.

And so we continue
        the myth.

Ode to the Thumbs

A stubborn belief
          in survival
was the seed
from which you sprang;
               naked, of course,
                         but not unarmed,
you became
          the final member
                    of the quorum,
and as the dissenting member,
you complete
          the hand.

All of humankind's progress
is based on the fact
          that you exist,
where you exist,
and that you did
          not evolve as just
                    another finger.

A new language
was invented
the day you arrived.
          All the statistics
          and percentages
          and histories
were then changed
          in your honor
in a quiet ceremony
          that no one
                    fully understands.

Because you exist
          outside the circle
you make it what
          it is; nothing less,
                    nothing more,
always first
          in line

for the many surprises
I have constantly
     warned you about.
You are the odd
       one out –
but you always
       come around
to the opposite point of view.

You have been known
    to build churches and chapels,
     both large and small –
but that just means
    you like to
      work together -
   as if harmony
     was a verb.

Looking at you
I realize
there will
    always be
      a quiet quest
      in your name,
always a question
     waiting
     for your approval,
a book of sand,
an ancient method of
    counting clouds -
   and a reason
     to finally stand alone.

Ode to the Fingers

I can sit
and watch the alternatives
        come and go;
they hesitate on
        the threshold,
then leave silently,
the smell of feathers
        and sliced air lingering,
but you still remain.

Tied to the end
        of an unfinished journey,
I accept you for that;
the thought of even beginning
        without you remains
too far in the distant past –
obscuring everything
        beyond my reach.

You of the mysterious
                origins
        and untold stories,
you arrange
        the random chaos
                of my life
        as best you can,
you divide the world
        into unequal parts
because I tell you to.
A segmented accomplice
        to my outlaw diaries
        and my outlaw ways.

But I can never grow
        beyond you,
you who taste
the earth in my name,
even when you are
        sheathed in my various
        gloves

and golden rings.

You speak for us,
you speak volumes
        without even trying.
We communicate with
        you and your
                secret language –
the one we all
        understand
                so well.

You help us tell
        our story
        with your
                digital precision
        and effortless beauty.
And you proudly wear our many
                status symbols -
                mostly on full display.
You act in tandem,
        the
        complete ballet –
you literally write
        the story of
                our lives.

Together -
        a wall of the
        first dimension,
a flight of
        digital geese;
the keeper
        of a thousand scars -
and, as I understand it,
        the final judge
        of all counted sums.

Ode to the Index Finger

To you we have
given the most terrible
        of responsibilities:
the first human touch,
the official seal of approval,
or perhaps not,
the path of
        one person's vision –
        only many times over.

And apparently
we have made you
        the final arbiter of our decisions,
both jury
        and judge,
always pointing
                to the victim
        of our wrath –
        or the recipient of
                our affection –
depending on the lighting
                in the room.

In your subtle manner
you became both the father
        of infinite detail,
and the son of our promise
that someday we
        will touch perfection,
that our hands will
        not tremble when we do,
that the night
        will circle back,
shedding the earth
        like an eagle,
that it will desire nothing,
                and never land.

Ode to the Third Finger of the Left Hand

That ring you wear,
there is a reason
            behind it.
A line of
            winter geese
swinging like a pendulum
            to the south;
            that is one of the reasons.
Seagulls wheeling
into the summer face
of an island sunset
            however briefly;
            that is a reason.
The black ravens
            of winter:
            they are also reasons.

Separated from
            the rest,
and reluctantly made
a symbol
to be looked upon
as a major course of action.
Either that or
the particular sequence of
            those certain rings that
                        you choose to wear.

Rings made of silver and gold –
            and occasionally small
                                    diamonds;
it has been said that
            marriage joins
                        power with beauty,
that the proportions
            are always exact,
and that change
            is a luxury
                        few can afford.

Mirror of the
        fragile season,
the season we are
                most vulnerable.
When you are naked you are
only useful
        to a single person,
the nameless soldier
        of the
                singular wars
we wage every day.

Encircled,
you become the
        promise of
                future generations –
        the ones only you
                        can see.

Ode to the Palms

Your face is
          crossed with
the tracks
          of a wild animal –
and although we deny it –
it's the one that we have all
          seen in our dreams.
The records
          of your birth
have been
          lost to us,
but not your purpose;
among other things
          you are the
          only cup that
                    I actually own.
And I cannot deny
that you have
          brought me water
          when I needed it
                    the most.

Soft harbor
          of my compassion,
when I hold things -
                    it is you
          who holds them
                    for me.

The first
          and last port
                    of our personal gifts –
both given and received -
          you are the ambassador
                    of our compassion -
          and those pleasant surprises
called life that
          we so enjoy.

Land of infinite

                    small ridges
and cryptic lines –
the ones telling us
of our past and
            the ones showing
our future in real time.
Apparently,
            you were the first
                        fortune-teller.
And all this time
            I did not know that.

You exact your toll
            on everything
                        you touch,
and everything,
                  in turn,
leaves it's unique mark
on you.
You enhance our
            ability to explain
our many passions in life –
and for this we
            are always grateful.

Gentle nest,
in your small world
            nothing
                  remains untouched:
the echoing of
            a song,
the small hand
            of time,
and snowflakes made
to last forever;
only these
            cannot
                  be given.

Ode to the Knuckles

Between you
ride all the important symbols:
      power on the right hand,
      beauty on the left,
and somewhere,
      somewhere near
          the border –
where knowledge
is direct and
      comes in waves –
you have found
      a home.

Hinge of small proportions
      and hidden openings,
you shape our verbs
      on a daily basis
      to your dimensions,
to your view
      of the universe –
and what you are
          asked to do
      on a daily basis.
And I specifically admire
      your ability
      to bend along the curve
of every handle
      ever known to humankind.
You easily learn
      the essential grip
      that we need
to master the demands
      of our time –
and our position
      in life.

I have not forgotten
the pain that sleeps
like a small volcano
    within you,

nor the scars and
        bruises that have covered
your wrinkled face -
as if the whole truth were
        a splash of red paint
                or a purple stain
that we reluctantly acknowledged —
and that we did this
        almost every day
                of our youth.

You give form
        and sequence
to my rhythms;
        to my book of
                sudden impulses.
The sum of your parts
is the definition of
        our shared memory.
Our list
        of past events
        that we cling to —
the ones
that always become our path
                        to the future.

And, as usual,
we await your response.

Ode to the Fingernails

We have reached
         an agreement,
         you and I,
I will be
         the tradition
and you will be
         the ritual.
It is hard to imagine
         us as being
         anything different,
this arrangement,
on another planet perhaps,
but on this one you became
         mother of pearl,
         rising slowly above my
curious fingers.
You represent the domestic talon
         and you have a life
                  of your own.

The various tasks
we put you to
         are beyond addition.
And how many times
         during the day
do we use you
         without recognizing
the patience of
         your growth
or the violence
         of your sudden setbacks?

Depending on your owner's
         whims
         you make opal
and other precious gems
jealous
         on a daily basis.

Painted one,

with your pale
>moon
>peeking out,
you give the world
a quiet update on
>our earthly status
at every turn.
And, according to
>our records,
you have worn these
>many masks
>and disguises
for millennia.

You, sheet of
>living mica,
formed from our daily
>events
and all of the strange sounds
>that they make.
The
common spade of the
>centuries,
>and the painful beginning
>of shovels.
How many tons
>of dirt —
>both rich and poor —
have resided,
>however briefly,
beneath your ragged roof
>these past eons?

You enter our lives pale,
>the flame already
>cool,
an ember glowing pink
and white,
and then,
brittle with age,
>you enter another dimension.
You become the

living map of
        our life-long endeavors.

You always mark
        the spot.

Ode to the Neck

With you
        no one had
        to start over.
Volcano of the
        supple island
we call home:
the sanctuary,
        the canyon and
        the dark cave
                of sound.
All the words
        ever spoken
have emerged from
        your depths,
words that
        can divide or unite continents,
words that touch
the softest skin,
or the darkness between
        the galaxies,
or no one,
        or nothing at all.
A parable
        of words,
        with your twists and turns,
        with your muscular pillars.
flexing to meet our every
                        purpose.

You knew why
        we were born
        before we did.

Spinal pathway and
        final station
                of our flexibility —
you and I have started
        so many journeys
        of a thousand miles
        with a single nod

that I have lost count –
but I know
          you have not.
As a word in itself
          you appear to
          have ninety-nine
                    lives –
and each one is
          slightly different
          from the last.
Early on you became
a sculptural concept
          that we are still trying
                    to understand.

Depending on the
          direction
                    you move,
you express our yes
                    and our no
with equal clarity
                    and urgency.
Your center of gravity,
          composed of migratory
bone and
arterial subways,
is at the mercy
of my vagrant eyes,
          like cattle rustlers,
scanning the horizon,
          the cliffs and
                    the rising rivers.

Deliberate avalanche of bone
          and tendon,
of unbroken flesh,
pedestal of the
          pivotal moment,
with your movable
          equator,
I celebrate you.
I circumnavigate

you with shells
        and leather,
with red stones,
and the damp
        velocity
                of longing.

Ode to the Back of the Neck

Everybody is
        doing what they
know how to do best,
and either getting better
        or worse at it,
and now when I
        look at you
it appears that
        the moon is the one
        causing the sunsets —
and not the
        other way around.

Erotic distance,
        the hidden chord of the
                cervical piano,
wearing a cloak
        of soft down,
sweat
and the lightening
        that is cold
        beneath the skin.

A silver mist
        enters the city,
swirling up the
        empty street,
I cover you
        in wool and leather
                and then I walk
                to seek the warmth
                of her fingers.
You embody the
        sensual world —
        wrapped in
smooth muscles,
        fine hair
                and erotic dreams.
I can't think of anything else
        but you at this

late hour.

The moon is falling now,
and time is receding
                into my past –
like the ghost
        that it is,
and here,
        my wide-eyed
        orphan of the
                lunar curve,
here,
        the warmth begins.

Ode to the Adams Apple

I cannot stop you
        from climbing
                your vertical tower,
nor count
        the steps
you take each day.
There are too many.
        Some are intentional,
some not.
It is all yours:
        the name,
                the meaning,
the difficult
        knowledge you carry within,
you who have witnessed
our most vulnerable
moments
and yet stayed
        with us —
waiting for either
        the beginning
                or the end:
        a topic we need to discuss
                        you and I.

Shield of
        living ivory
        and sudden movement —
you protect our
        verbs and nouns,
                poems and arias,
you determine our
        personal resonance,
                you shape
                our musical paths -
                both short and long.

Rising into
        the wind like
        a singular falcon

with your
unique signature –
as if you were
a thief who steals
only from the
      anonymous,
or a machine
that performs flawlessly
and cannot
      be explained.

Swallow,
      cliff-dancing swallow.
You dance
      your singular dance
as you explain our position
      in life,
as if you had
      a choice,
or a say in the matter,
      or your two cents worth,
as if the
      whole world
was watching.

      You take me
          with you.

      You dance.

Ode to the Bones

We are tied
        together
you and I.
You shape me,
and I,
I move you
with my myriad
        muscles,
my many dreams,
        and my determined destinations
both near and far –
sometimes not far enough
and others
        that reach over the
                horizon.

Ribs, cranium,
elbows, you
exist in the
nouns we have
        reserved
for structural purposes.
Hollow in nature,
with your antiseptic
                core,
consumed with
        movement
                and strength
in your mute and mostly
                blunt way.

Enough,
        you will
                never be enough,
but you will
outlast me,
and I must
remember that,
now, while it

                    still counts.

You have
          sculpted me
from the beginning,
stretching me taut,
          like a relentless
                    mechanism,
programmed to
          grow in miniature
          and mostly mathematical
                              leaps.
With your slow
          correctness and
something bordering on intuition
          and fate
           you have already
decided how
I will look
          to the world.
And you take such pride in
the values you've assumed:
          rigidity and substance,
perseverance
          and a certain
                    directness –
          which I openly admire.

Living stone,
wrapped in
dark red strands,
          you grow
          in minute ways,
you slumber
          without sleeping,
while steadily building
your engineered
          intricacies,
your skeletal bridges.
          And you do this
                    while living,
mostly quietly,

beneath our
     flesh.

So stay with me now, please,
    and, yes, remember me,
       in your special way,
      when I am gone.

Ode to the Marrow

Inner core:
all richness
and no glory, no fame,
      silent and
      sealed in your
         living shell,
     no heartbeat,
     no breath,
but you keep
     us healthy
to the best of your
         abilities.

Birthplace of a
      billion miracles
every day,
complex matrix and
      cellular factory
      you are the silent fountainhead
that feeds our veins
      and arteries
      with life itself –
and you return to this
      task every second
        of every day.
And, apparently,
     you are quite
      the poet.

We try to support you -
with our unreliable
      lives,
our uncertain expenses and
expectations,
     our near daily substitutions -
and every night we ask your
       forgiveness -
which you quietly
      give.

I think I can hear
        you sighing
                when you do.

Mute battlements,
and inner defenses,
you guard
        our medical shores,
with your minute marines,
with your white
                warriors,
and your red warriors,
sailing,
        ever sailing
the bloody and
        rushing main.

We've always needed you.
        We just have
        strange ways
                of showing
                our appreciation.

Unseen one,
        submarine one,
        our lighthouse of good health
lying just beneath
                the soft waves
that we call beauty.
        We thank you
for your song,
        your aria,
the one we hope to listen to
                        forever.

Ode to the Joints

You extend me,
        with your defined
forms and simple, singular intentions.
And my world is infinitely larger
because of you.
How could I move
        without you?
You who cup my hands and
give meaning to movement,
        any movement,
all movements.

Each of you,
individual,
        and set in your ways,
you are sometimes stubborn
                to the extreme,
but when you work together you give us
        a symphony
of laughter
        and dance
                and so much more –
                        a living and
                        immediate ballet
                                of sorts.

And I am the sometimes
haphazard and infamous
        conductor
of our personal symphony,
        leading you
constantly into darkness and uncertainty -
        often unprepared.

I admit that I
am reckless at times,
but you have given me this:
        a certain freedom
        of movement,

116

and now I demand
        nothing less.

Twist, bend,
        touch, turn;
these are
        your verbs.
Run, jump, leap, reach;
you give meaning
        to these words as well.
Throw, catch, thrust:
I depend on all
        your pivotal qualities,
on your ability to
        bend to my will
at the precise moment,
the moment
                at hand,
and the movement
                intended
for some greater glory -
or perhaps
        a quiet life –
yes, a life in harmony,
as in, sometimes we do
        not have to
defend our
        every move.

And when we grow older,
        I know you will complain,
sometimes loudly,
about my many poor choices -
but I will never blame you.
        At least we have that
        understanding between us.

We are in this together
        you and I,
                and to the end.

Ode to the Face

For every emotion,
        you require
        an outward gesture,
the center stage, so to speak,
being the echo
        of our soul,
being the fountain,
        the pool,
and the reflection all at once.

You have taken it
        upon yourself
to convey our personal images
of strength or beauty,
        or sometimes both –
and you have succeeded.
Your meanings are found
                in thin layers
        and your layers
                are infinite.

You are the owner's manual
        of our impromptu response;
hieroglyphic,
        cryptic,
                enigmatic,
these are also
        your names,
as if you alone invented sculpture,
        or the distinct footprints of smoke,
                or even symmetry itself.
Painted map
        and cryptic lighthouse
        of our moods
                and inner meanings.
You give fair warnings
                when needed –
which we often ignore.
And I'm fairly certain

this is something
                       we need to discuss –
sooner, and then again
                                later.

You are the
the first and final
                 sacrifice
         to our gods of beauty.
You are both the bookkeeper
and the mask
        of our lives.
Our personal mask,
the one we tend to,
and then try to erase
                every day.
And occasionally we
           succeed.

You write the lines
of our slowly gathered wisdom
onto our pliant, waiting face
with a steady hand,
on a daily basis
         mostly in silence,
behind the walls we build
              against the wind.

And then,
        with your blessing –
              we continue.

Ode to the Jawbone

Wearing your mantle
            of silt and
                        petrified light –
or was that really ivory?
And now listed variously as:
            the beginning of
                        anthropology,
the trajectory of black whales,
            or the mandible of a
                        carnivorous angel:
The one who was not quite
                        a saint.

Gateway
            of our unsatisfied hunger –
                        mostly when circumstances
                        spin beyond our control,
with your necklace
of sharpened pearls,
dull stones
            and your small lodes
            of silver and gold,
you move to rhythms
as basic as the waves
            of our planet.
And you have always
            stood for something
                        bigger than yourself.

Torn between falling to the earth
            and our most elementary needs,
carrying the white daggers
            of hunger in your belt,
you guide our
            pirate ships
toward the richest ports available
            in our multi-colored world.

And in your wake;
            only the bones.

Ode to the Chin

Made of wheat,
        eagle feathers,
                and every rock
known to humankind,
you define all
        the principles
of a lifting body
or the physics
        of individual love or,
perhaps,
        something in between.

You became the spring-board,
        the place to start,
the place we can build our
                fantasies upon.

You set the stage
and then we stack
        our faces upon you.
We play out
        our comedies,
our dramas
        and tragedies,
and we hand you
        the mask
and then you draw
        the one line
that defines us.

We use words
        like snow,
night, reflection, love, birth,
sunrise, sunset,
        and story,
                my story
                        your truth.

And then you
        draw the line.

Ode to the Mouth

Such a small
        opening
through which
we pour the fruits,
        the grains,
        and the various beasts
of our labor;
in our need
        you refuse nothing –
at our pleasure,
                all.
Vital entrance,
        portal of thirst,
hunger and those other
measures of luxury
        that we can
                sometimes afford.

And yes, I realize that
the number of words
        to adequately describe you
        and what you do for us
        would fill the pages
                of several romance novels
and, possibly,
        a small dictionary.

So I will use you,
        sculptor of our words,
carpenter of our
        verbal responses.
With you I will shape
        the inquiry,
the long communication,
the dance of winter,
        and the silence of the wind
                beyond the horizon.

I am going now.

I will wear you
    like a
    small constellation.

Ode to the Lips

Small orbits
of flesh,
alternately
        hot and cold,
I can sometimes read
        ecstasy
between your lines.
And sometimes sorrow –
        and for the same reason.

Delicate red stones,
living stones,
you are the keepers
        of our secrets,
bleeding into the wind
with your silence,
arriving quietly
        in my dreams,
then rising slowly:
that and the setting
                of sails –
they are often
        the same.

You talk to
        our souls
when you are
        aroused,
you bring home
        the trophies.
Sound-maker,
        you can read
        between the lines
and play every
        instrument.

Occasionally symmetrical,
        sensitive and delicate –
our hopes

             and occasional dreams flow
easily through you –
you are a better
communicator than
our words by themselves.

You are the navigational aide
             of our infancy –
and then you continue
             in your exploration of our
             intimate worlds and travels
             as they spin before us. .
Apparently at some point
             in time you became
                          an archer
of impressive skill.
             Your arrows are small
             but generally accurate.

And finally,
             have we discussed the concept
             of fullness?
I think that
             is the hidden conversation
that we'd all like to have with you
                          some day.

Ode to the Tongue

Most of the time
I keep you
        in the dark,
and you wait,
        impatiently,
and when I
        let you out,
like a mischievous elf,
you invent a life
        of your own;
waving my dreams,
        my hopes and fears
like tattered laundry
to any passer-by.
But sometimes
you give me
        the pleasure
of giving pleasure;
        and that is
                your gift in return.

Interpreter,
        harvester,
                and daily gatherer
of our salt and honey;
the final judge
of what is ripe -
        and what
                must wait.

You live your life
        in the shadows,
always hoping
        for a reply
so you may again emerge
from your dark cage.
And for you
        it is always
                a question of timing.

Ode to the Teeth

I came upon you
        unexpectedly,
you were growing quietly with
        a whiteness
stolen secretly
        from the swans.
At first I could
        not tell if you
were serious about
        staying;
you would fall away
        at odd times
leaving me with a
red hole here and there
        filled with pain,
        completely useless,
but then,
        phoenix-like,
others would
rise in your place
        and stay,
without promising –
        just staying.

And so I put you
        in charge of my life –
my everyday life,
ivory enigmas,
living stones
        pitted with
                my trying existence,
from the irregular
        holocausts
of bread and meat
        and the occasional means
to wash them
                down
in some kind of style.

I've always had an
          estranged relation
with you – starting
          with endless dentists
          staring uncomfortably
at your seemingly
          haphazard arrangement
                    in my mouth.
They thought we had
          some type of
                    agreement.

And so I keep you,
          and so you keep me,
in this stylistic contract
                    of sorts.

You, flying in
your ancient
and practical
          formation –
like dental geese,
returning to
          the southern shores,
the resonant coasts,
and now to
          the harvest feast.

You anticipate abundance
                    of course,
and occasionally
          I can deliver.

Just don't get
          used to it.

Ode to the Nose

Let us hasten,
            you and I,
until we meet
                        halfway,
until the world
lies at our feet –
            ripe and filled
                        with enormous odors.

Let us celebrate a
planet of individual smells,
            pungent smells –
and you,
            a net of fine hair
and delicate nerves
poised to capture
            our primal urges,
                        our necessities,
            and the many olfactory
             pleasures we seek –
seemingly without end.

Let us turn
            into the ethereal day
as if you were
            a hooked beak,
and I a bird of prey.
Let us seek out,
            you and I,
the vast olfactory banquet
that lies somewhere
            beyond
                        the open gate.

Sculptural event,
            nasal wing,
            facial pier of sorts;
someday
I will shove you

into a
        circle of flowers
and abandon you.

But for now
let us hasten,
        you and I,
until we meet at the crossroads
        of sense and the
                        sensual.

Today let us
bait our traps
to catch
        the unseen –
and the elusive vision of how
        our lives will
                really be.

Ode to the Nostrils

I will call you
the gift of waiting,
   the belated concern,
   the equine fold.
You in turn
   will give me
your unhurried gaze,
   a gaze more vivid
      than sight,
remembered as
   the time when,
      the place where,
         the person her.

Twin dolphins,
   matching the colors
of the nautical wind
with your olfactory answers,
   filling your sails
with the billowing
   smoke, dust and odors
of our singular
   domain –
the domain we agreed upon –
   as I remember,
      after much debate
      and many miles.

You touch my days equally,
   yet you choose
   from them
only a handful of memories,
   a passage here and there perhaps,
that and the slow turning
      of the fragrant -
and sometimes forgotten pages –
   also known
      as memories:

The ones we keep
      hidden in our pocket

Ode to the Eyes

Here is where
      light begins.

This is
where you announce the
      emergence of the world
             to us.

You are like
      no other organ,
fluttering sometimes,
lately of the
      morning winds;
you pull the shadowed forms
and colors into focus.

You are where
      the new begins
           every day,
the dawn of
      color, hue and tint.
You are
      the recorder of our
      intimate, and otherwise, secrets,
quiet center
      of the storm,
camera,
      camera,
           movie,
               movie
and, yes,
      map reader.

You are both the beauty
      and the beholder,
jury and
      judge,
invitation and
        reply.

You are the
          distance closed,
the molecule
          uncovered,
the horizon,
          always
          just within our reach.

Being small
water-filled worlds,
and having so much to do
with pain and pleasure
          and their many translations,
places, objects,
and more
          explanations,
until finally –
we have explained
          everything –
          and we are
                    blind once more.

Here is where
          light begins.

Ode to the Pupils

You gather every
        crumb of light
                that falls within my reach
like two shining
        black ants,
and you carry
them back
        to the center
                of my being.
And you store
each speck
        very carefully,
now because
        it is spring,
now because there
is such a thing
        as winter,
now because
        the darkness
                will come
                        again.

Black hole surrounded
        by hands of
        brown, sapphire
                and green opal,
the sun, moon,
        stars and earth
step into your hands
and you lift them
        into my life,
        like an   elevator,
with your doors
opening and closing,
squeezing and crowding
        every ounce
                of light
that you can hold
into an opening

                    so small that
only trees, mountains,
                    distant lovers
and small planets
            can pass through.
You do this
      because you know I
            will never see
            enough to soothe
                    my restless soul.

Ode to the Eyelids

Thin shell,
       living shell
meant to block or chase
       the sun;
the semi-automatic shutters
       of our mind.
Quick and slow,
       often fringed and painted
              like a reclining orchid,
delicate shield of skin;
you stand
       between us and
the angry winds of this world,
       the infinite dust,
and the many sights
       we'd rather
              not see.

Pale water boy,
you bring the moisture
       that glistens and soothes;
you hasten the beginning
              of tears,
you smooth the way.
You earn our respect
       every single day –
as if we can't live
       without you.

Sometimes I forget
       that there are two of you –
and that you always meet
              in the middle.
       I like that arrangement.
It's something I think
       we should continue
              if we can.

You are the brave home of
    eyelashes and sweat,
        paint and glitter.
And often,
    more glitter.
And yet you rarely complain.
Caretaker of our tears,
    we also entrust you
        with our secrets
and you keep them well.
        Sometimes.

Close friend,
you are there when I
    need you,
you blink,
    and then we continue
        our intimate journey.

Ode to the Eyelashes

Star sweepers,
       sleep catchers,
              dust stops;
our linear collection
       of mostly useful hair.
If we could –
       we'd grow more
           of you –
we're just not sure how.

You line the eyelid
like a declaration
       of many nations,
while the sun
       glints copper,
              topaz and azure
along your
       willowy shores.

Buried beneath mascara
       you have been
            a tool of beauty
for many women
       for many years,
            for a mostly singular reason.

Umbrella of sorts,
you defend our eyes
       from the flying sands
           and sparks
of a wind–driven,
and sometimes angry world,
with your short
       vertical bursts
and your graceful
       parabolic curves.

At night
       your gentle fingers

meet at
       mid-vision,
closing at
       mid-desire,
signaling either the
violent release
       or the sighs
       and silence of dreams.

You comb the
air until
       it is mostly clean.

You divide
the light itself
as if you were
       a knife
              of silken feathers,
passing as
       quickly as
              the shadow
       of an eagle
              beneath
              the mid-day sun.

Ode to the Eyebrows

Our vestigial
                    crest
has receded,
          now wisely lying
flat along
          the forehead,
just beyond
          the fire's reach.
A simple analogy;
and then the sensuous
          incident
          is remembered.

You display the
          sweat of our labor,
          our forward radiators,
a cool breeze
becomes your purpose.
We break away and
          then go on
and on a good day
          we can run
                    forever.
That was my latest dream
                    anyway.

Plucked and
painted,
you draw the
          beautiful line,
rising like a
          crescent moon
above the iridescent eyes,
you become the edge
          of mascara,
the beginning
          of beauty,
and the exotic dance to come.

All form evolves
          after the first
                    definition,
after the first blows
                    of reality
                    set in.

You were
          only a matter
                    of time.
And now it is enough
to know
          that you were born
                    with wings in mind.

Ode to the Forehead

Weathervane
    of the minutes,
            the emotions
and the dark fears
    of the day,
you wrap
    your wrinkled hand
just above the brow
trying faithfully
    to reproduce
            the rare image,
    the glimpse
        of motion,
the solemn understanding
    of what it means
            to be free.

Broad riverbed
    of wisdom,
        sadness and concern,
you bend ideas
    into arrows,
you roll back
the elements
    like a wind-driven ship.
And sometimes
    you approve
    of my trying ways.

Visual sum
    of our striking advantage,
silent,
    and mostly smooth volume
        of reason,
you knew you were the means
    to an end.
And that you always
            have been.

The ticking
        of the clock
gently touches you;
it feels like
        warm rain
        and the night,
the one
        we agreed to.

Ode to the Cheeks

Soft invention
and second beginning,
          supple cheeks,
you grow the
          facial garden –
blooming and fading
          with our various seasons
                    and our daily tasks.

You wave the flag
          of our emotions.
And oftentimes
          we can see
                    our heart
                    through you.
You've always
          had trouble
          hiding our
          innermost feelings.
But you keep trying.

Traffic director –
          you also make sure
                    we don't starve.
You water
          the garden.

As the day closes,
          dragging it's
                    glowing feet
behind the clouds,
you are there,
          vibrant,
                    restless,
                              impatient:
Waiting to start anew.

Tonight you
smell of roses,
          goat's milk

and thistles –
and I have no idea how
           that happened.

Home of
        stray hairs
        and various shades of ruby paint,
tranquility
        and contentment,
        famine and hope,
you write the book
        of our lives
on a daily
        basis –
        with your wrinkles for words –
and you always make sense.

You claim to be
           the ultimate matchmaker
and I know you well –
        you would wed me
                   to the future.

Ode to the Temples

Aerodynamic wedges,
      co-pilots,
      you cling to
           our heads
like decals
      painted onto
      the sides of pure velocity,
that
      and the will to survive.

As I understand it,
      you are more
          myth
      than reality.
You live on
      a line
between the eyes
      and the ears
as if you were
      born to dance
on the edge
      of a cliff,
      always on the edge
and,
      because of this,
you will never change,
and you will never
      grow old,
      one way or
          the other.

Opium den,
      I can descend
into your smoky depths
by stroking you
      with my weary fingers –
that and all the
      time it takes.

Beneath your
        supple façade
lie the mysteries
of this world
        and our memories
                of those worlds past.

With my fingers
        I can unlock your wisdom,
I can unravel
the infinite
        additions
that we call
        our days.

And today I will
call you wealth –
        and then
        I will spend you.

This, so that
I may see you again
                tomorrow.
That –
        and all the time
                it takes.

Ode to the Mustache and Beard

The reasons
            are simple enough;
to look better,
            to look different
to remind us of who we choose
                        to become
                        at any given moment.

            The
            virile manifesto,
both haste
            and laziness,
and also history –
and all the other myths
            we'd like to think are true.

Soft
            and wispy,
or bold and rugged
according to
            your history and heritage,
and sometimes certain genes;
and you become the honest
                        referral of our inner selves.
            At least for the moment.

Your meanings can be
                        infinite –
as if empires
            and grand entrances
were only one hair
among your thousands.
And now I'm starting to realize
            that forever and
            the end of my life –
                        are the same thing.

You have been braided
            and ribboned,
curled, perfumed and waxed

by the finest
          warriors
                    of our many clans.
The clans who keep
          our past.

And a pirate,
          you are like a flag
to be raised
          or lowered
according to our moods,
our various seasons
          and latitudes.

You itch and tickle,
you give rashes to
                    our loved ones.
You collect dust,
          butter and stew
                    in equal portions.

You know that
you are generally
more trouble than
          you are worth
but as you have also known
          for quite some time,
our vanity will
          dull the razor
                    faster
                    than any rock.

Ode to the Ears

This is where the waves
      enter,
with their aural
      colors, chromas
          and intensities,
and you,
      somehow you understand
         these mysteries.
      And you keep trying to
         explain them
              to me.

Cranial flower;
      I can trace
         your convolutions
back to our shared quest
         for knowledge
         and human survival.
And, I'd say we've done
      fairly well
         at that.

You call yourself
      outer, middle and inner —
as if they were separate earths
         and those other
         intriguing myths
      you would have us
           believe.

All
      ridges and valleys,
you channel your
      reality
      according to our
         latest choices.

You guide us
through the darkness at night,
      and in the light

we bejewel you,
and hang
        our various gold and silver prizes
from your supple handle,
        and you usually agree,
and then
        you guide us -
                again.

You contain
        the treasure
                of balance
somewhere deep
within you,
somewhere among
        the flats
                and the sharps,
the tremolos and
                progressions;
and all the many musical treasures
that you willingly share with us –
                if only we will take you there.

"Aye, captain",
you say,
        here,
        where the
                waves enter.

Ode to the Earlobes

This is a musical
                subject
        for some reason –
and a subject worth
            mentioning
I might add.

I know this is true
because I have listened
        to the bells,
the chimes,
            and the seashells
            tinkling with the wind,
or the slow turning
            of her head,
as if these earlobes
were the most
            delicate of birds –
and that our life
was gentle enough
        to permit us
                to hold them.

These are the
            precious treasures
that we give you,
            earlobes,
and in return
        you
        give us your
                many pleasures.

Hanging there,
        looking very much
        like a butterfly
                about to emerge,
I can trace
        your sensual path
down to the
        fertile soil

153

and then back again;
you complete
       the circuit.
And why are you
       so delicious?
And why do I
       want to kiss you?
I think we deserve
       some answers here.

Sometimes
       I think
you were
       a hindsight,
put there to keep
       the ear
from spinning
       off our heads,
or perhaps
       a bauble,
put there in a
       moment
          of celestial laughter.

But I also believe that
       you are real
          and meant to be:
At night
you leave the taste
       of wax and sweat
          on my tongue.

Ode to the Hair

Yes, if you are
      long – you flow,
but
      more than that;
you open every sensory gateway
      I can think of.
You light the darkness
      with your dancing,
you suffer our vanities
      and then return with
          your brilliant results.

You've known these things
      for some time now;
that somehow
      you influence
      our loves,
          our actions,
      our sorrows and
          satisfactions.

No one asked
      but you replied
          by growing,
by curling,
by coming and
      then going.

You become the gilded
frame of her
      face
      at mid-night,
the crown of light
that she wears
on sun-filled days
      and other special occasions.

You move like the wind -
slowly rippling across
          the ripening field,
and then
          coming to rest
          on our heads -
with your
          unshakeable faith,
your sincere
          belief in our
                    tomorrows;
and your premonition that
          we will cross
                    many bridges
while looking for
          our home.

Ode to the Voice

You create the hole
        when all we see is ice,
vibrating in your
        many frequencies with our
        every thought
                and feeling –
        more than we can count, really.

Unfortunately,
        we occasionally experience a
        spontaneous flight
                of many short words –
and many times I regret
        knowing you as well
                        as I do.

You thrive as the
        unique fingerprints
                of our souls –
        because you speak
                        as each of us,
                yet your voice is
        always distinct,
        and sometimes –
                you are equally distant.

But if I listen closely
        you tell me that
I am with either family
                and friends,
        – or my daily cast of
                total strangers –
        depending on today's
                        errands.

You change
        like a green chameleon -
        according to our moods
                our opening scenes –
and often from scripts
                written by others –
that we would surely
        like to know.

You are
        muscle and tendon,
                marble and clouds,
        past and present –
and me always trying
                to catch up.

You are both song
        and the reason we can sing.
You are the gateway to
                hello and good-bye
        and all of the many emotions
                that come in between.

And, yes,
        you have asked me this
                        before.

Ode to the Lungs

If we set out to
describe
     the only person
we could ever love,
I'm sure we would
spend the rest
     of our lives looking
          for this person.

Believe me,
it is much better to let
them describe
     themselves;
     they are so much
     easier
          to find
          that way.

I feel as if I
     am a satellite
revolving around you,
     my lungs,
and yet you cling
     to me.
You feel
like a new leaf,
     wet from the rains,
young and full
     of life;
and you know
it is your mission to succeed –
     that life exists within
          your careful hands.

And you do.

But so often

I have been cruel to you.
Which you have accepted
                    for so many years.
And chances are,
            you will never
                    forgive me.
I know this.
            We will talk about
                    this tomorrow.

And you:
            supremely honest;
you ache
            when I push
                    too hard,
too fast
and that is basically when
            I know you the best.

And you and I?
It seems as though
            we have
reached some
type of agreement;
and I realize this
            when you are tearing
                    great chunks of wind
from the high Andean air
like some pink
            and carnivorous
                    bird of prey –
because this is
            where we are.

And here's something we can
both live by;
            I will race you
            to the end of
                    my life,

if you will fill me
          with precious breath
                    for the rest of yours.

Ode to the Liver

Vital organ,
we need to
      come to an understanding,
you and I.
      A truce -
            a vital pact if you will.

If we review
our history together
      it seems like
I have been at war
         with you
for most of
         my life.
And I confess that I
      have not been very kind
         to you these
            many years.

Lucky for me,
      you have not
         surrendered;
you know
      that I cannot survive
without you.
You have
      known this
         for a long time.
And it is a secret
      we are happy
         to share.

Blood red,
      living filter,
a visceral vacuum
      of sorts,
you clear the path ahead;

we send you
       our daily poisons,
              for better or worse,
and you confront them
              straight on,
       and you generally
                     prevail.

You have become the dark place
       where most of our daily secrets
begin
       and end –
and you know that.
       And you feel rightfully
                     proud.

Our metabolic armory;
       you store our
vital supplies,
and then you return
       them
              daily –
as needed,
       and, mostly,
              just enough.

Promethean gland,
in spite of my daily abuse
you regenerate;
       you keep coming
              back for more.
And I am forever counting
                     on that.

So tonight let us begin
       the vital negotiation
              once more;
       so that I may live
              to greet you again
                     in the morning.

Ode to the Throat

Passage,
the muscular slide
     to the stomach,
segmented
     and simple:
all ribs and cartilage,
     home of the larynx
and various other
     useful exits
     and entrances.

The receiving dock
for our comestibles
     and combustibles,
for our precious oxygen
and many other
     less-rarified
        elements.

You sort the constant
     incoming
        barrage.
You channel the
     threads of life
that weave their way
into our every nook, pore
     and cranny
until we become
     the living fabric
of our own culinary choices
or the lack thereof –
and our place at the
     human table.

There is a beginning
     and endless

                        quality
about you:
the voice shaper,
          the shaper of our words
and songs:
our invisible handshake
          with the world.

You are the first
          to taste who
we have
          become in life,
rich or poor,
– or trying and perhaps
          somewhere in between.

And then there
is you and I
          and our very singular agreement,
and then passage,
              passage,
                  always passage.

Ode to the Stomach

Now,
        take a dam
        made of hungry fingers,
for example.

Ode to the Intestines

Both a large and small drama,
and a
        a process akin
to life itself.
You feel
        like a familiar ritual,
like something I've
done many times,
        and, mostly,
                to perfection.

And usually I have
        your cooperation
as the proud owner of
this order of things
        that I can never really
                change,
        even if I would like to.

You know quite intimately
our current standing with
        the world –
our status and
        our vital statistics.
You always have the
        final say,
                or so it seems –
and then, of course, you throw in
        the occasional
                surprise or two.

At times
you've been more
        stubborn than
the proverbial
        mule.
You have your

                own direction
that you cling to and
you seem to
           take some pleasure
in disagreeing
           with me in
           the strangest of places —
and usually quite
                remote.

And when times
are plentiful,
           you take
more than you need,
and I have known
           few times that
we did not
have to pay
           in some small way,
some shy glimpses
           missed,
some small perfection
           compromised,
perhaps a
           bridge
                uncrossed,
a bus ride untaken,
a warm smile unseen -
           all because you called me
           at the worst possible time.

But somehow we survive,
           you and I.
We need each other,
           sometimes desperately,
                and, yes,
I'll always forgive you —
                as if I had
                    a choice.

Ode to the Kidneys

Fraternal twins,
         our personal pair of back-yard pyramids
             and other eastern mysteries.
You invented
      osmosis.
Yes, osmosis itself,
so many eons ago,
and thankfully,
      you still
          own the patent today.

A pair of
      metabolic beans,
      you keep an eye on
so many of our personal things,
intimate things,
      and the things we can't
          live without.

In a perfectly timed
      hormonal dance,
an exchange
      of precious enzymes,
an understanding
        of urine,
and a balancing act
      of infinite
         proportions –
who we ask
      for your daily help.
And, often,
      for your understanding.

Renal filter,
      royal filter,
you filter our daily

                    rituals and habits.
You know every secret
          we've ever tried
                    to keep.
And we listen to you.
          Mainly because
                    we have little choice:
          You are both the rock
                    and the hard place.

Ode to the Glands

Collectively,
you form the
        endocrine cartel;
you produce
just about all of our
        natural resources.
And then you often hold us
            for ransom.

You built the home
        of our hormones —
the ones we really need,
and you became generally
        symmetrical in your
            responses
to our daily excursions —
            both short and long.
You provide the balance
        in our lives
that we often
        don't know
            we need.

Silent sentries,
you seem
        to have
all of our bases
        covered,
both coming
        and going.

        And growing.

I guess we're lucky
        that way.

Ode to the Appendix

I never really
       met you,
but now I am glad
       you are gone.

Tiny, ticking
       time bomb.

Ode to the Blood

I guess you know
me better than I do –
     and you always have.
You've seen
     every part of me,
         every day
more intimately than
     I could ever hope to,
and there is
     something awe-inspiring
in that.
Something I will
     never fully understand.

There is nothing
about me that
     can live
         without you:
the common link,
the ancient
     lineage,
     the family connection –
         and our scattered
            family clan.

You touch everything
about me:
the yearning for symmetry,
     the awkwardness,
     the obsessions,
         everything.

Coursing through
my face, arms and legs
following your
     predetermined path,

both delivery boy
      and garbage man,
the stream itself,
         the proverbial medium of life.

Your redness
      is legendary
and is the favored liquid of poems,
         prayers, promises,
         and all the other heroic tales.
You wrote the Iliad
      in your sleep.

You point out
      the obvious,
the shared secret,
the secret of all living things,
      and should we lose you,
      we lose everything;
you write
      our most intimate contract
         with this uncountable world.

And we always sign
         on the dotted line.

Ode to the Veins and Arteries

You carry the
        heart's beat,
the pulse of
        vermillion and red,
and the teeming life
        therein.
You conspire
with the miles,
        and you have
mapped my existence
from the beginning,
from the ancient
        fingerprints
of my ancestors
to the many seas
        within your small blue channels.

You send and receive
        the warm surges,
the semaphores of
        my flagship,
                my body,
signaling every inch
of my existence
with
your tree-like
        branches
extending
        to every leaf,
to the smallest of our countless leaves.
This, apparently, is your
        daily objective
        a goal taken
                seriously.
Even when it rains,
it is something

you seem
       to care deeply about.

Supple aqueducts,
       with your one-way turnstiles:
both coming and going
you advance
       our civilizations
against every
       struggle
through your small openings,
and you have
       never questioned
              that purpose,
your existential mandate,
your personal
              directive –
and something we've shared
       forever it seems.

Path seekers,
the ultimate conduits
of the human
       condition.
And all of your paths
lead to the daily market:
       you supply the demand.

Ode to the Skin

Pale covering,
red, brown, black covering,
    earth-born hues,
echoing all of the colors of
Mother
    Earth's own
        thin surface.

Smooth, rough,
moist, dry,
also describe
    your varied terrain,
your ever-changing
    topography.
the soft lesson
    of human expression.

You change!
So what shall I
    call you today?
Do you have a
name for each
    of your textures?
You go by only one name –
    but how can that be?
I can see that you
    have many faces;
each one different,
each one
like a mirror unto itself,
coming from a
    different reflection,
a different place
    or a different name on
        the human map.

Fragile covering,
you are knit of
      delicate strands
that can stretch
      to accommodate
      the most gentle
or the wildest of our moves.

But you also have
      your limits;
I have lost count
of the scars I have
      collected
      from my careless past,
and our many encounters
      with the concept of velocity
and the honed edge
        of everyday life.

And yet you
      are still calm and
            unafraid,
quiet,
supple skin –
      even knowing that I
        have not
        changed my ways.

Ode to the Wrinkles

Wrinkles,
I know what
      you mean,
and what you bring:
      a rose that
      you found a
            long time ago
and somehow preserved.
And now you've
      brought it
            to my door.

So come in!
I can't deny
      that you are standing
there,
with retreat
      in your eyes,
an innocent
      smile on your lips,
and that damned rose.

So tell me,
      my little friend,
      where shall
            I wear this one?

Ode to the Smile

Little smile,
you turn
        the saddest tide,
you lift the
        corners of my mouth,
of my entire world really,
        you ease
all the sharp edges
        of this universe
        and, mostly,
                the ones we least expect,
as the reminder
        that we must
                be brave enough
        to see the truth
and then be the ones
        who live it –
        one way or another.
You mark the beginning
        of our inner selves,
you know how to communicate
                without words,
you spawn dimples
        without even thinking –
                it is simply your nature.

Your hidden talents include
pleasure,
        old friends,
                happiness,
        joy
                and amusement.
You pave the sometimes
        rocky way
                to laughter.

Light-switch,
          wisp of muscle
          and lips,
          a slow upward curl
                    of caring,
medicinal
          and magic;
you can
          heal the
          unseen wounds
and soothe
          the unquiet heart.
You can lift
          years from
                    a troubled face
with your simple appearance
                    at center stage.

As a gift
to someone new
          in our lives
you become
          more than
                    precious:
you continue the meeting,
          you seal the deal,
                    as the yeast of friendship,
and the bread made of
                    personal bridges.

Among those we
          know well,
you signal the
          joyful remembrance,
the bright pennies
          of our concern,
and the soft hello
          from our heart.

You spring easily from
everything that
              touches us.
Your roots are
              found in
the five senses:
              the heart,
                      the mind,
the ironies,
              the pleasures,
                      and the predicaments
of the human
              condition.

And the small
                      things,
the ones
              unforeseen,
the ones least planned,
              and often,
                      the most welcome:
              the little
              waif that accompanies us
across the bridge
              of memories –
                      the memories
                      we want to keep.

Ode to the Brain

We started something
a long time ago
without really
        knowing it,
                you and I.
But now I can't
        remember when.

And it continues.
Sometimes I
wonder if you
are really a part
        of me;
often you seem
                beyond
my reach and
        unwilling to listen,
stubborn at times,
        reticent
                at others.
Mostly you seem
        to be controlled
by vagrant urges,
        earthly desires
                and erotic dreams –
                anything but reason.

Words:
        you invented them.
So is it possible
to describe you
        with your own words ?
Can a mirror looking
        into a mirror
ever really
        describe itself ?

Grey realm
        of the intellect,
bustling depot of arriving
        and departing
                neurons,
command post
        under almost constant siege.
Legion
        are the images,
sounds and smells,
        both coming and going,
and legion your responses —
you process them all —
                sooner or later.

Cluttered, chaotic
        post office
                of the psyche,
sometimes
        I wait months,
                or even years
        for a reply from you.
And it appears
        that some of those
                letters
are lost forever
amid the confusion,
the constant deluge,
        the junk mail
                and the cheap shots.

But I do get
        my replies,
        eventually,
postage due
        or not —
        and then,
usually,

something about

        return to sender.

Ode to the Heart

Well, we've come
      this far,
            you and I.

I suppose
      you already know
that you are
      the center
of my world,
and perhaps
that makes you feel
      a little smug.
It should.

Life force,
      unsleeping one,
seemingly
      without end
      you go on and on
and you
take me
      with you.
And I
      gratefully follow,
intimately tied to a muscle
I know will
      someday
tire of its
      constant toil
      and my added insults.

You rely on shadows
in order to be seen,
and yes, I hear
      your constant complaints;
they are not lost

on my vagrant ways
and my
     frequent
         indulgences.
Adrenaline meter,
you measure my
     fear or my fatigue
even if they have
     passed,
and quite accurately
     I might add.

Do you also measure
     my love
         for another?
Yes, yes you do,
     and very well
         at that –
I can hear you quite clearly
     when she
         enters the room.

Blind and
     unthinking,
you obey commands
that I have not given
     and can rarely
         control;
and it is one of
     your many virtues that I
         constantly count on.
And I continue to count -
     because you have
         so many truths.

By my reckoning:
         at least
         one for every
             day.

Ode to the Body in Motion

I guess I have
      seen you
            enough times,
and in so many places,
in an endless profusion
      of activities.

You should be
      familiar by now,
            but you aren't,
and perhaps you
      know it:
a constant presence —
      no matter what I am doing.

You are my familiar one
yet my mind refuses to
      believe that
your infinite
      displays
of grace,
      agility,
            and control
all come from
      the same body,
my body,
      the same supple machine
given to us
      with careful instructions
to explore
      every inch,
cover every distance
      and achieve every height
            within our grasp.

And somehow
        we have succeeded
through you,
        in spite of you,
                because of you.

Living container
            of motion,
the embodiment of
                constant change,
you move in every
            direction at once.
Even when
        you appear outwardly calm
your inner waves
        never cease —
crashing constantly against
        the shores
                of our intimate time.

Aye, aye my captain,
        my sailor,
                and my ship:
now be my ocean,
        let us sail anew
        each day
on the endless sea,
now let us continue
        the dance,
        the endless motion.

Ode to the Body Asleep

Small, quiet breaths,
these are the silent rhythm
            of our
            sometimes restless sleep,
when we choose the
            nocturnal statues,
and our many poses
            of our flight into darkness:
our nightly
            departure and return.

Sleep
            is slowly sifting
through the leaves
of our limbs now
            like a warm tropical rain
and we are still,
            becalmed,
                        and waiting,
gathering up the
            mist of our dreams
in preparation
            for the dawn
                        and the hunt
for the oncoming day.

Body asleep,
            the keeper of dreams.
Our dreams are like the
            ocean waves –
            no two are ever the same.

            You show us the
                        the innocence of sleep,
and the secrets
            that we try but

                    cannot share.
This is our time
           of healing,
the time of the rejuvenation
of our physical
                       village,
this renewal of
our will to live –
           and then to live well.

Body asleep,
pausing briefly
in a state of
           splendid singularity,
as our mind
escapes to the
           many dimensions
                       of our dreams,
some real, some not –
           this mysterious
                       duality
that we cannot live
           for long without.

The minute flickers
           of our muscles,
and the sudden jolts from
           another world,
some imagined,
           and some not,
the slow, languid
           glide of a
tanned arm as it crosses the pillow;
these are the familiar movements
           and the cryptic ballet
                       of sleep.

So for now
           we will dance again

               my friend.
It is late.
        I am tired.
And let us be honest
        for a change:
               it is our favorite
                      time of day.

Ode to the Body in Sickness and in Health

We ache,
      you and I,
sometimes I know why -
      but not always.

You seem to find
all of these lost and orphaned
diseases and then
      you bring them home.
      And you adopt them.
Your hospitality is
      endless,
and my decisions
      are often less than brilliant.
I won't even mention
the innumerable
      cuts, bruises, burns
         and abrasions
from my foolish childhood
      and my careless adulthood
that you have somehow endured.
      But this is no time
         for jokes.

There doesn't seem
      to be a single
part of me that
      is not susceptible
         to something –
something you have tried
      to warn me about
but I have mostly ignored.
Often there is
      no cure,
      and sometimes
         little hope

for what we get
        ourselves into.

But you, body,
      are my constant
         warrior,
with your microscopic armies,
with their antiseptic swords,
      and your unceasing
         vigilance,
         and mostly gentle cures.

And who trained you?
I see no medical
degree hanging
      on your wall.
So how am I to believe you?
But then I think:
      there are so few others
         I can turn to
      in these uncertain days.

There is something
      magical about you,
something I hear
      from within,
words spoken to me,
words of wisdom,
      words spoken
         by a trusted friend.

There is a quiet resonance
      between us
and we know it,
and I find strength
      in your song.

We are tired,
      we ache

you and I,
and then we start again.

Ode to the Fat and the Skinny, the Tall and the Short

There is more
        to it,
than just pounds –
        or the lack
                of them.
A view of my knees
        is nice –
        but it's not everything.
Looking around,
we think some people
        have it made –
until we've seen it all
and then
        we're not sure
                it's all that important.

It is.

We make it
        our business.
We see to it
        that it is.

We sneak glances
        in the store windows
        as we walk past,
we listen to the voices
        as we leave
                the room.
We admire from afar,
        or snicker, or stare.
We measure heights –
                or not,
        with each encounter,
and it determines how
        we conduct most

of our daily excursions.
It even appears,
  occasionally,
    in our voices.
We are aghast at
  the extremes,
but the standard
  is forever changing –
and the finger is
  forever wagging.

We both admire
  and pity
those who can
accept themselves
  as they are –
for they have
either won or lost
  some magnificent battle
    from within.

And the rest
  of us?
We will continue
  the struggle,
    perhaps forever.
Because, you see,
  there is
    more to it
    than meets the eye.

Ode to the Cycles and Seasons

It's that time of
years:
the lunar
        timeline,
and the terrestrial
        velocity,
the golden spiral
        of the ocean nautilus,
we spin to you,
        and then we turn,
and turn
        again.
I am constantly
        amazed at your
        deep understanding
of the word circadian
        and that you live by
                its rules –
                every single day.

All points of
        the compass
        are your
                captives,
the rising of
        the sun
is your starting point –
no matter
        the season;
we play to you
        and we sing,
and then we sing
        again
no matter the day.

And we suffer,

alone,
and suffer with
            our own,
because you
      will not
            be stopped —
and they will understand why.
The obvious
      continuum
of your soul,
your pride is
      discussed in
blooming flowers
      and then,
            equally,
                  in falling
                        leaves.
Our
      daily
            archangel,
your seasons,
the endless
      belief
that tomorrow
      will come -
and that we will take
      the calculated risk
                  to go on.

We are
      always with you,
a life-long captive of your
      comings and goings,
and, hopefully,
we will be
      with you
            tomorrow.

And then we awake,
    and
      we begin again.

Ode to the Death of the Body (Requiem)

We come to it
      suddenly –
or perhaps with great
      forethought –
and we leave with –
         or without –
the approval
of those we
      love –
      or, occasionally, those we hate.
To adoration and
      parades,
or the single tear,
      or perhaps
         a knowing laugh as
we leave
      this earthly world
for the home of our private
      gods,
or, more often,
      places unknown
         and unseen:
because we know
that death is
      the final silence.

We fight,
often with quiet
      elegance
or loud
      determination.

We cling,
we swagger
      and lie,
we gnash our teeth,

we lock our
            doors
and turn
         our eyes,
and then
        we hope
for the best —
        while always fearing
               the worst.

We enter this world
        in grace and innocence,
with no
        remembrance
of the past
        or fear
of the future,
        and we leave
        with an abundance
              of both:
like tin cans
        tied to the tail
           of a cat -
          running for
              our lives.

Ode to the Birth of a Child

The tiny
          fist,
strong beyond
          its days,
the parents
          pride,
strong beyond
          their years;
a cosmic, unexplainable
longing
          now fulfilled,
a new journey
          just begun,
with all the bridges
          soon to be built –
          and then burned –
and then built again.

At this particular threshold,
          the long shadow
                    of uncertainty looms.
At first
          hesitant,
the sails slowly
                    unfold,
little one,
and then we see that you
                    have just begun.

You step
into an unlikely,
          and often unwelcoming,
                    world.
You have
          emerged,
mostly defenseless

and dependent,
with your
seemingly endless needs,
and we shall try to
answer them,
one by one
if we can –
if you will
let us.

The cage
has opened now,
little eaglet,
and you have flown –
and now there is no turning back.

You will
never return to us
completely,
and we have known this
from the beginning,
but always,
we hope,
that you will circle
near.

The Last Goodbye (The Love Poem)

Goodbyes are for
                strangers
and passing acquaintances –
not for friends
         and definitely not for
                        lovers.

Spoken or unspoken,
         the last goodbye
              is always:
                        I love you.

About Atmosphere Press

Atmosphere Press is an independent, full-service publisher for excellent books in all genres and for all audiences. Learn more about what we do at atmospherepress.com.

We encourage you to check out some of Atmosphere's latest releases, which are available at Amazon.com and via order from your local bookstore:

I Would Tell You a Secret, poetry by Hayden Dansky

Aegis of Waves, poetry by Elder Gideon

Streetscapes, poetry by Martin Jon Porter

Feast, poetry by Alexandra Antonopoulos

River, Run!, poetry by Caitlin Jackson

Poems for the Asylum, by Daniel J. Lutz

Licorice, poetry by Liz Bruno

Etching the Ghost, poetry by Cathleen Cohen

Spindrift, poetry by Laurence W. Thomas

A Glorious Poetic Rage, poetry by Elmo Shade

Numbered Like the Psalms, poetry by Catharine Phillips

Verses of Drought, poetry by Gregory Broadbent

Canine in the Promised Land, poetry by Philip J, Kowalski

About the Author

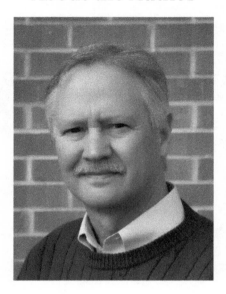

Born and raised in Idaho, Joe currently lives in Boise. He earned his Master's degree in Architecture from the University of Idaho, practiced architecture in Idaho and California for over forty years, and taught architectural design at the U of Idaho for nine years. Nowadays, Joe enjoys being retired and free to work on personal creative projects, including raising an annual vegetable garden and "playing in the dirt."

Joe was introduced to the poetry of Pablo Neruda while living in Santiago, Chile many years ago and that is where the idea for writing the Odes was born. In addition to Pablo Neruda, Mother Earth and Nature have always been major sources of inspiration.

CPSIA information can be obtained
at www.ICGtesting.com
Printed in the USA
BVHW070336060821
613732BV00006B/654